Jean
Melanson
604-858·2363

RAIN ON A DISTANT ROOF

RAIN

ON A DISTANT ROOF

A PERSONAL JOURNEY THROUGH LYME DISEASE IN CANADA

VANESSA FARNSWORTH

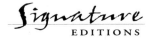
EDITIONS

Cover design by Doowah Design.
Interior design by Melody Morrissette.
Photograph of Vanessa Farnsworth by Peter McLennan.

This book was printed on Ancient Forest Friendly paper.
Printed and bound in Canada by Hignell Book Printing Inc.

We acknowledge the support of the Canada Council for the Arts and the Manitoba Arts Council for our publishing program.

Library and Archives Canada Cataloguing in Publication

Farnsworth, Vanessa, 1968-, author
          Rain on a distant roof : a personal journey through Lyme disease in Canada /
Vanessa Farnsworth.

Includes bibliographical references.
Issued in print and electronic formats.
ISBN 978-1-927426-23-4 (pbk.).—ISBN 978-1-927426-24-1 (epub)

          1. Farnsworth, Vanessa, 1968-, —Health. 2. Lyme disease— Patients—Canada—
Biography. 3. Lyme disease—Canada. 4. Lyme disease—Treatment—Canada. I.
Title.

RA644.L94F37 2013   616.9'246   C2013-905431-6
                                                                  C2013-905432-4

Signature Editions
P.O. Box 206, RPO Corydon, Winnipeg, Manitoba, R3M 3S7
www.signature-editions.com

dedicated to
Dr. N. Richard Pragnell

for leading me out of the hell
that others led me into

*He began: "What fortune or what destiny
leads you down here before your final hour?
And who is this one showing you the way?"*

— Dante Alighieri
The Divine Comedy

CONTENTS

PART 1: INFERNO

Give up all hope of ever seeing Heaven:
I come to lead you to the other shore,
into eternal darkness, ice, and fire.

— Dante Alighieri
Inferno

A RURAL MYTH

For most Canadians, Lyme disease is more of a rural myth than a reality. It's a disease that exists primarily in rumors or the kinds of magazines that squeeze medical oddities between ads for miracle diets and million-dollar salaries that can be earned from the comfort of your mobile home. The average person has never met anyone with the disease but, if they stretch their memories, maybe they can recall hearing that a brother of their cousin's ex-husband's father may have had a buddy whose niece once had it.

Or maybe that was lupus.

In January 2007, I knew what just about everyone knows about Lyme disease: That you get it from being bitten by an infected tick and that it makes you sick in some vaguely defined way. It's possible I could even have told you that it was named after the town of Lyme, Connecticut, one of three neighboring communities where in the mid-1970's the children fell ill in what appeared to be an outbreak of juvenile rheumatoid arthritis.

Only juvenile rheumatoid arthritis doesn't come in outbreaks.

One of the funny things about Lyme is that more people can tell you where the disease got its name than its primary symptoms. Still, I wasn't thinking about Lyme disease or ticks as I slopped through the dirty slush on my way to the dentist's office.

I was in a purple mood.

After thirty cavity-free years, I suddenly had two that needed to be filled.

I resented the inconvenience. I resented the expense. I resented the slush.

Like I said, purple mood.

I don't know what I expected when I sat down in the dentist's chair, but I imagine it had something to do with staring blankly at unadorned ceiling tiles while trying to ignore the sound of the drill. The good news is that the drill is in no way memorable. What is memorable is what happened when the dentist shot the freezing into my gums.

I started to fall. Through the floor. Through the Earth. Out the other side of the planet. Heat blasted up my spine, setting off earthquakes in my legs. Fear exploded like a grenade. This didn't strike me as a normal reaction to a simple shot.

It didn't strike the dentist that way either.

I said, "Allergic reaction?"

He looked dubious.

I pressed down on my legs as hard as I could, but my arms weren't strong enough to contain the tremors so I gave up and instead turned my attention to determining whether it was physically possible for the procedure to continue. It was, although the dentist had to stop every thirty seconds because I was dogged by the sensation that my tongue was being dragged backwards down my throat.

How many years ago was that? Too many.

And yet the sensation that I'm on the verge of swallowing my tongue has never gone away.

Things quickly went from bad to worse.

Of course they did.

There wouldn't be a story if they hadn't.

In the days following that fateful dentist visit, I would develop a staggering number of symptoms in addition to the ones that erupted in the dentist's office: a runny nose, headaches, vertigo, diarrhea, aching muscles and joints, fatigue, nausea, weakness, disorientation, a racing heartbeat, shortness of breath, blurred vision, insatiable thirst, anxiety and fainting spells.

These symptoms were unstable, abruptly arriving and departing as though a series of switches were being flicked on and off by a wizard hidden behind a curtain. One minute, I'd feel as though I had the worst flu of my life and the next I'd have no symptoms at all. Then moments later some or all of the symptoms would reappear.

Those awful kaleidoscoping symptoms.

If I'd written them down at twenty-minute intervals, each record would contain a unique set of data as though I were a nurse strolling through a ward, challenging myself to recall what was wrong with each one of my patients. Sometimes the lists would overlap — even lightning occasionally strikes twice — but in most cases the symptoms recorded at 1:30 p.m. would have nothing in common with those recorded at 2:00 p.m. except that they were all manifesting in a single human.

It was complete chaos.

There seemed to be no rhyme or reason when a symptom would appear or disappear and nighttime was the worst. Fevers would ascend just after sundown, causing me to swing violently between thermometer-melting highs and shaking chills until the small hours of the morning while waves of energy pulsed through my body. There were times when my spine would get so hot that I'd lie on my stomach for fear that the sheets would catch fire.

And I really did fear that.

Because the fevers brought the crazy with them.

I wouldn't know where I was or I'd believe I was someplace I'd never been. The Taj Mahal. Maybe Seville.

I had nonsensical conversations that I addressed to no one in particular.

If my husband asked me a question, I'd give him an answer that had nothing to do with the question he asked and I was powerless to do anything about it.

"Are you okay?"

"The wind is causing the snow to blow upwards."

"It isn't snowing. What are you talking about?"

"You can see both of them if you close one eye."

"I don't understand."

"There aren't any chips left."

"What's the matter with you?"

"Blue."

As I was saying this, I'd be watching the air pleat before my eyes like curtains slowly being drawn and stars falling from the ceiling. And I'd be shoving tissues up my nostrils in an attempt to stanch the bleeding that would otherwise have forced me to sit up or change position, neither of which would've yielded positive results.

Those fevers. You could set your watch by them. They'd arrive at 10 o'clock every second night and fade by 3 a.m. the following morning. German trains don't run with greater accuracy.

I'd never before encountered a fever that operated on such precise 48-hour cycles, transforming me into a wild-eyed human ember one evening and leaving me mercifully fever-free the next. So free that I'd think the febrile stage had passed and surely this strange illness was taking its leave. Only then the fever would strike again the following night like a hostile employee arriving promptly on schedule.

But who or what was setting that schedule?

And what would it take to get them to stop?

I've learned a lot since then and one of the things I've learned is that much of what I've described above is atypical.

This is not how Lyme disease is supposed to begin.

Just ask an expert, if you can find one, or a public health official, if you can't. And if you live in Canada, you probably can't. Trust me, I've done the legwork on this one and I can tell you that trail leads nowhere.

While I was at it, I scanned pamphlets, studied books, scoured research papers, read case studies, and, occasionally, queried those whose area of research or clinical expertise led me to believe they might be able to answer my questions. This is how I know that Lyme disease is supposed to begin with a tick bite followed closely by flu-like symptoms that can include fatigue, chills, fevers, headaches, muscle and joint pain, and swollen lymph nodes. There can also be a rash which, depending on the source you consult, manifests in between 20 and 80 percent of all Lyme cases. Yes, that's a wide range, but if you've had Lyme for as long as I have, you get used to so-called experts disagreeing — sometimes quite vociferously — over each and every aspect of the disease, including the prevalence of acute-stage rashes.

And these rashes are important.

The one that crops up most often in Lyme disease literature features a series of concentric red and white rings that taken together look very much like a large, slightly misshapen bull's eye. Photos of this rash show up so often in official information about Lyme disease that you'd think it's a common manifestation.

It isn't.

It's so cool that it brings out the voyeur in doctors and civilians alike, leading them to read a monograph on a disease they would otherwise pass over on their way to more relevant illnesses like cancer or diabetes.

When present, this bull's-eye rash is diagnostic of Lyme, but the early-stage rashes associated with this disease often look more like nebula or like white stars with red coronas. Sometimes a rash takes the form of a big red blotch that looks very much like someone dipped a sponge in acid and pressed it to the skin while at other times there are multiple bright red blotches that bring to mind lily pads strewn across the surface of a pond. My favorite looks very much like an embarrassed fairy ring — clear in the middle with a bright red rim.

But let's forget about the specifics for a moment.

When can be as important as *what* when it comes to Lyme symptoms. That's another interesting thing I've learned from reading up on this illness: You run the greatest risk of contracting Lyme in the cool months of the year when young ticks are most active. May has proven to be the most popular month for acquiring a Lyme infection, but you have a realistic chance of picking one up anytime between April and July or in the autumn between October and December.

Conventional wisdom says you don't catch Lyme in the dead of winter.

And you certainly don't contract it from a dentist's needle.

But all of that is trivia.

I don't recall a tick bite and my skin has never played host to any bull's eyes, lily pads, fairy rings, nebulae or stars with funky coronas. If I'd ever seen anything like that on my body I would've freaked.

I did freak.

These freak-outs just had something other than rashes at their core.

At least they did at first.

When I showed up at the emergency room one Saturday morning soon after the strange illness began to manifest, it was a busy place and the doctor on duty had no time for medical mysteries.

Illnesses run predictable courses.

Symptoms don't flicker on and off like fireflies on a warm summer evening and even if they did, there were far too many symptoms spanning all systems of my body.

Only a crazy person would make the claims I was making.

And I felt crazy. I felt truly insane.

I was being told that the illness I was describing wasn't possible and yet I was sure I was describing it accurately.

It's not that the doctor didn't give me options. He said maybe a virus, maybe the early stages of multiple sclerosis, maybe a thyroid condition, but he felt it critical to emphasize that he was leaning towards crazy and so should I.

I left the emergency room wishing I had lied, wishing that I'd known what lie to tell so that I would've gotten help instead of being shown the door. In order to have done that, though, I would've needed to have some idea what was wrong with me and tailored my story to suit the diagnosis I was looking for. But I was completely at a loss. I had no clue what was wrong with me.

Then one day, a week or so after the fevers arrived, they abruptly stopped. For good, I thought.

But no, they would return again a few weeks later and repeat the distinct 48-hour cycle. Then, finally, a month or so after the strange illness began, a switch was flicked and the symptoms that had been plaguing me suddenly vanished.

That's where this story should end.

Instead, it's where it begins.

A HARD SELL

The roller-coasting fevers are gone and so are the flickering symptoms.
And yet I can't shake the feeling that something is horribly wrong.

Nor can I point to a defining symptom.

All I can do is note that something inside me has fundamentally changed and not for the better. It occurs to me that I may be dying; that in some dark corner of my anatomy an important cluster of cells has charted a fatal course and one day soon someone will slap a name on the illness that's siphoning off my life.

A doctor.

Possibly a coroner.

Who am I kidding? The dogged pursuit of causation truly exists only on television dramas where characters have more curiosity, energy and charisma than those of us who exist in the real world. Here everyone is too tired, too overworked, too distracted to put any real effort into determining the cause of anything. I'm not sure what the medical term for "who knows why you're sick?" is, but I'm sure it exists.

Idiopathic comes to mind.

Maybe that's why heart failure shows up in so many obituaries. Ultimately that's what we all die of anyway. I mean, you can be completely brain dead, but as long as something — your native heart or a machine that functions much like it — is pumping blood through your veins, you're still technically alive.

No pumping, no life.

And since we, as a society, have been primed to believe that sometimes hearts simply stop beating all on their own, we accept that as being a legitimate cause of death without putting too much thought into it.

Dude died from heart failure.

Too bad for dude.

But I'm getting sidetracked.

It's now been several months since the fevers and the merry band of symptoms they brought with them abruptly decamped, but now my reproductive hormones seem to have gone haywire. My periods now last for twenty days out of every month and hot flashes drag me out of bed in the middle of the night to wander the house naked in the hope that the night air will chill my skin.

I fantasize about sleeping in a freezer. I debate the merits of being frozen like a goldfish into a block of ice. I punch a wall.

My mood swings are as unpredictable as they are violent. This morning I was crying inconsolably over a crack in a vase that five minutes earlier I'd forgotten I even owned. At noon I was giddy to the point of agitation over a million-dollar windfall that was promised to me in an unsolicited email from some African country I barely knew existed and by mid-afternoon I was so hyperactive that I couldn't concentrate on any one thought for longer than a second.

And now?

Now my legs are finding movement irresistible.

I'm pacing around my office like a caged tiger, thoughts giggling through my brain until the most illogical one clicks into place and I find myself on the verge of doing something only a cartoon character would consider reasonable.

I'm not going to tell you what. It doesn't really matter what.

I'm crying again and I don't have a clue why.

Actually, I do have a clue why. Something is in control of my emotions and it isn't me.

I run all this by a doctor.

Perimenopause, I'm told.

I look around for something to throw. Messengers rarely make out well at times like this.

I argue that 38 is hardly old enough for perimenopause to be settling in, but the doctor disagrees and I don't have any solid evidence to refute his diagnosis. I only have wounded vanity and a nagging feeling that there's more going on here than a natural part of the aging process. But the nagging suspicions of a patient mean nothing to a doctor, so efforts are taken to stabilize my hormones and I try to convince myself that at the ripe old age of 38 I'm being dragged helplessly into menopause.

It's a hard sell.

I consult that compendium of reliable medical information known as the Internet and discover that if I use a well-greased shoehorn, I can coax most of my symptoms into the wonky hormone category and the ones that don't fit can be ignored.

And I discover to my great relief that I don't really care all that much about aging.

All I care about is sleeping as many hours as I can.

I care about this passionately.

Soon 12 hours grow to 16 and during the brief time that I'm technically awake, I'm so exhausted that I spend my time counting the minutes until I can crawl back into bed and sleep some more.

I'm about as functional as a grizzly in December.

Even breathing seems to exhaust me and digesting food depletes my energy to the point where I have to nap after meals.

If I'm slowly morphing into a bear, I'm doing so with imperfect results. Grizzlies enter hibernation in the autumn and lumber out of their caves in the spring.

I'm doing the opposite.

But then I'm new to this.

Even so, I'm looking forward to hibernating for months on end in the hopes that the extended down time will knock the fatigue right out of me and then everything will return to normal. I try to convince myself that I believe this and discover, to my great chagrin, that I'm not as gullible as I was hoping I would be.

I live on a rural property in southeastern British Columbia, which means, among other things, that in order to fetch my mail I have to dodge potholes and deer and the occasional self-liberated cow as I struggle down the dirt road to the cluster of mailboxes out on the main thoroughfare.

So when a fluffy orange dog trots towards me, I'm hardly surprised.

That's not to suggest I'm in the mood for all that fluffy orange cuteness, because I'm not. I'm too busy regretting my decision to go for a walk to do much more than notice, then ignore, its existence. My hip feels like it's blown a bearing and the pain is rapidly disabling my leg. If I had a marker, I could draw the path the pain is traveling, starting in my lower abdomen and ending at the tip of my big toe. Actually, I'm not sure it really ends there, but since I don't see any sparks shooting out the front of my boot, I'm going to have to take it on faith that the pain dead-ends when it hits the edge of my body.

Or possibly my aura.

I'm going with my aura.

My hip didn't hurt before I set out on my mail-retrieving mission, but now that I'm a quarter of a mile from home with no choice but to hobble all the way back, it's decided to mess me up in a major way.

I guess that isn't really all that surprising. My left leg has been getting increasingly difficult to move over the past several weeks to the point where if I try to swing it forward in a simple walking motion, it refuses to obey my command, so in order to take a stride, I have to kick it backwards and swing it in an awkward semicircle. My lower back is left to do all the hard work, so by rights it should be the first to complain, but instead my hip decides to steal its thunder.

Weird. Exhausting. Totally messed up.

I'm sure I look odd when I walk, but there's no one around to see me except for the fluffy orange dog and I'm ignoring him. If he so much as places his paws on my thighs, I'll topple and spend the next half hour trying to figure out how to contort my body into the right position so that I can struggle back up.

In truth, more than my leg is acting up. All of my limbs feel as though they've been sewn on backwards, so whenever I try to roll over in bed or maneuver around an obstacle in my path, I get all tangled up and have to expend a ridiculous amount of energy figuring out how to untangle myself. This is particularly annoying because I'd mastered all this by the time I was three, so why am I not the master of it now?

I don't know the answer.

What I do know is that I absolutely don't want to fall over, so I stand post-still and eye the dog's distracted approach. He pees on a tree, noses around in some weeds, then bobs his head in time to a passing butterfly. When he spots me he starts to trot, only to be caught short by a sudden puff of wind, and all I can think is, "I know this dog." The main thing I know about him is that he's inseparable from his owner, so I look past the dog and determine that his owner is nowhere to be seen.

I tilt my head, but no, he's not lying in the ditch.

The fluffy orange dog has evidently done a runner and it occurs to me that I should really know his name since it's the same as my husband's, so being able to recall that bit of trivia and yet not be able to break out a name is a bit distressing. I'm stumped, or I would be if I weren't suddenly distracted by an odd twinge in my chest. Something has grabbed hold of my heart and is squeezing it like one of those rubber balls people use to relieve stress.

My heart is suddenly the only thing I can hear. It's beating at half its normal rate. No, it's beating much slower than that. It's beating so slowly that I can sense immortality between each labored thump.

The dog starts to spin and so does the road.

I rise like helium. At least I feel like I do, but considering I'm not actually gaining in altitude, it must be just a sensation.

It occurs to me that half of my heart is no longer beating and I wonder which half as I flutter my fingers against the dog's bouncing head, trying to distract myself from the idea that if I move too quickly, my heart will stop beating forever.

I stare up at the clear blue sky and concentrate on taking smooth, slow breaths.

A dozen or so beats go by before my chest again twinges and my heart returns to a normal rhythm as though nothing has happened. And still I stare at the sky, afraid to move, not having a clue how I'm going to get back home.

I wish I could tell you that this is an isolated incident, but it isn't.

There are times when my heart beats so slowly that I'm certain it's going to stop, and always I freeze, afraid of what will happen if I dare to move or cry out.

A doctor tells me that whenever this happens I should go to the emergency room.

Sometimes I do, but mostly I don't.

The problem is that by the time I arrive at the hospital, the crisis has passed and no one is quite willing to believe that a perfectly healthy, possibly menopausal, 38-year-old woman could have a serious heart condition.

Because in their minds, perfectly healthy is what I am.

I don't get a vote.

But I do get lectured. I'm wasting everyone's time over what's likely nothing worse than palpitations or esophageal spasms.

Hypochondriac. Take the crazy with you when you leave.

ROCK BOTTOM

It always amazes me how far down rock bottom really is. This is as true for the medically doomed as it is for your average substance abuser.

The ache in my left hip grows steadily worse and, as the days stretch into weeks, the pain spreads to my spine and moves upwards, causing my vertebrae to feel pulverized and my ribcage to feel splintered. I could scream.

I do scream.

There's no position I can sit, stand, or lie in that doesn't leave me in agony. I no longer breathe so much as shallowly puff like a guppy in a fish tank.

Doctors continue to insist they can find nothing wrong with me. Their tests are telling them that I'm perfectly healthy.

I'm telling them that I'm perfectly not. I question the accuracy of their tests.

Doctors question the accuracy of the information I'm giving them.

We hit an impasse. A stalemate.

But the strange illness has no intention of forging any ceasefires. Symptoms are starting to snowball. Chills are swirling across the left side of my body as though a breeze has somehow become trapped beneath my skin and is growing increasingly restless. My spine is vibrating like a string on a harp. A strange tingling sensation is swarming the back of my head and my hands are buzzing like they've just spent hours operating a jackhammer and can't quite believe that the hammering has finally stopped.

It's now mid-May, more than four months after the mystery illness entered my life, and rashes are moving across my skin, one day showing up on my thighs, the next on the top of my feet, the day after that splayed across my nose and cheeks like a giant sleeping butterfly.

These rashes are driving me nuts. They come and go without rhyme or reason. And sting like vinegar-spritzed wounds. Nothing I try brings me any relief nor does anything the doctor tries, but he does inform me that the rashes are likely due to contact dermatitis, so whenever one appears I need to examine everything I've come in contact with so that I can identify the elusive trigger and dismiss it from my life.

Only I fail miserably.

These rashes seem to be self-triggering and that's the last thing I want them to be.

I'm staring at a doctor.

He's staring at me.

He has no intention of addressing a long list of symptoms and isn't afraid to tell me so. He's in a vile mood. Or maybe that's just his personality, it's hard to tell.

Anyway, the doctor demands that I pick one symptom and he will investigate that, nothing else.

But my problem isn't a single symptom, it's a growing cacophony of them, and a doctor who will only investigate one symptom is about as much use to me as an ice cube in Antarctica. So I pick one and wait for permission to leave.

From my perspective, my health is rapidly declining. Every system in my body is falling apart. I'm on a one-way trip to immortality.

That doctors see things differently has not escaped my notice. According to them, my rashes are the result of contact dermatitis and have nothing to do with the pain in my hip, the hormonal hiccups, the radically slow heartbeat, or any of the other symptoms that are elbowing their way into my body.

All of my problems are separate and inviolate. Or so I'm being asked to believe. That they all showed up in the wake of that odd illness in January is relevant only to me. From the doctors' perspective, I'm blowing things out of proportion. Connecting dots that shouldn't be connected.

So I stop reporting my symptoms to doctors. I'm tired of being told that I'm so healthy I could run a marathon. I can't run a marathon. I can barely keep my eyes open.

The tests are wrong. They aren't giving a complete or even an accurate picture of what's going on, but the only one who seems to know that is me. I no longer believe that perimenopause is the underlying cause for any of my symptoms and although I don't have a clue what is, the feeling that I'm dying is now reaching a fever pitch. And I'm at a loss as to where I can turn to for help.

I only know where I can no longer turn.

I have no idea how sick I am; that after months of valiantly fighting invading organisms all on its own, my immune system is finally losing the battle and the infection is spreading like a wildfire through my organs and brain, scorching everything in its path.

I won't learn this for many months.

The only thing I know right now — and I know this for certain — is that I've been handed a puzzle with a critical piece missing and I need that critical piece to turn up soon because I'm rapidly spiraling downwards with no bottom in sight.

In an odd way, it's almost a relief when I lose the feeling in my big toes.

They no longer hurt.

They don't burn or tingle or sting.

They don't anything.

They're absences at the tips of my feet.

Absences that I should probably do something about.

So I'm at the chiropractor's office, because for some crazy reason, I think she can fix this. You know, pop a splintering vertebra back into place and voila, my toes will light back up.

I tell her this.

She frowns.

"That's not a good sign."

"What is these days?"

"This isn't funny. You need to see a doctor right away."

"I've already seen a doctor. I've seen lots of them. Those conversations always dead-end with me being kicked to the curb like somebody's week-old trash."

"Still, you've got to try."

"Or what?"

"It's not my place to say."

"Evidently it's no one's place to say. That's how I got into this mess in the first place. No one wants to say anything other than I'm spectacularly healthy. As if. My toes have disappeared. How is that normal?"

"It isn't."

ONE FATEFUL DAY IN JUNE

Somewhere in the middle of the night things have taken a turn for the worse. I didn't think that was possible, but it seems that hell has more levels than I previously realized. I'm guessing this is level twenty or possibly even thirty, but I'll have to check with Dante on that one and get back to you.

Only not now.

Now my joints are aching and so is my spine.

I'm moving like the Tin Man in *The Wizard of Oz*, but at least I'm moving and that can only be a positive sign. By rights, I should be lying in bed whimpering like a wounded puppy, but I have a client who's eager to get his project underway, so I stumble out of bed, determined to make the epic journey from my bedroom on the second floor to my office at the far end of the basement.

It isn't easy. I'm hot and I'm dizzy. My feet ache with every step.

I switch to walking on my heels, which doesn't improve the situation in the slightest, so I settle on a flat-footed shuffle and grit my teeth.

Christ, my hip is useless.

That last sentence should be in all caps, but I'm too tired to breathe, let alone retype a sentence.

I make it down two flights of stairs thanks to the combined forces of gravity and inertia. Physics seemed so pointless in high school, but today, when I've got a buck to make and an engine that's running on fumes, these fundamental laws land my butt in my office chair despite my body's protests. And what more can I ask of physics than that?

Maybe it could also erase my headache.

Didn't think so.

The headache remains, but it does have one distinct benefit: It's now so painful that I've almost completely forgotten about the paisley rashes swirling across my thighs. Did I mention those? No? Consider them mentioned.

Work has been known to have the same effect — making me forget my problems, I mean — so I buckle down, knowing that once I immerse myself in the project at hand my ailments will become little more than background noise.

Only they don't. Heat and fatigue are dragging me down. I glance towards the rug, thinking how nice it would be to curl up on it. These glances become increasingly frequent.

My headache shifts into a new phase. It feels like the plates of my skull are fissuring and my eyes are so stiff it's hard to move them in any direction, so I rest them on the computer screen, which responds by flicking pixels at my eyeballs. Mercilessly. Endlessly.

Fine, whatever. Since it's clear that I'm going to accomplish nothing today, I decide to go upstairs and lie down, only when I try to stand, my legs give way and I find myself face down on a wool rug, napping like a child in nursery school.

And just like a child in nursery school, I'm restless.

The pain in my skull has reached Chernobyl levels and the heat is unbearable.

My thoughts are scrambled eggs.

Worse, my neck and eyes are locked in fixed positions.

If I wasn't in the thirtieth stage of hell before, I'm surely there now.

I wonder where my husband is?

Clearly not here.

I wish I had one of those signaling devices like Commissioner Gordon in the Batman comics. Then all I'd have to do is aim it at the clouds and kick back, knowing its lure to be irresistible. But I don't have a signaling device, so if I want to go up to the bedroom I'll have to figure out some way of getting there on my own.

I try to stand, but the walls sway and my legs caramelize.

Crawling it is.

"Crawling" might not be the right word, since crawling would be an improvement on what I'm doing, but whatever the right word is, it's painful.

And slow.

I navigate across the basement floor on my hands and knees and go up the stairs to the main floor the same way. Then I crawl across the living room floor to yet another flight of stairs and across yet another hardwood floor to my bed high up in the second-story loft.

This is all so unnecessary. There's a couch in the living room that I could've easily flopped on but, like a wounded cat, I seek out a safe place to hide while I wait on my husband's return. That safe place is my bedroom.

Once there, I lie on the bed and imagine that I'm a radiator sending up steam.

I do this for hours.

When my husband finally turns up, I'm too weak to call out so I tap on the wall above the bed in the hope he'll hear my signal. He does and searches the entire house trying to figure out where it's coming from, with the bedroom being the last place he looks.

He tells me I look like hell.

I return the compliment.

He pops a thermometer in my mouth and it posts a temperature of 40° C, but neither of us knows if that's high, so my husband breaks out the information sheet that came with the thermometer and gives it a read.

Forty degrees is high.

The pain in my head has now surpassed Chernobyl levels on its way to birthing a new star and I'm afraid that if I touch my skull, I'll discover that the plates have popped apart from the pressure and the heat.

My husband suggests that maybe swinging by the hospital might be a good idea.

Swinging by the hospital is never a good idea.

I've been to that emergency room enough times in the preceding months to know that my problems will be greeted with malignant disinterest and I'll be told:

a) That my illness, though manifesting in my body, is really all in my head.

b) That I'm overreacting to a simple case of the flu.

c) That emergency services are meant for patients more worthy than me.

I can't stand the thought of having yet another doctor push me out the door having done no more than the minimum the law requires. Or worse. To be faced with a doctor who has already failed me.

I decide to sleep the whole thing off, but my husband is growing increasingly concerned so he goes off to phone a nurse. He describes the stiff eyes and the even stiffer neck, the high fevers, the skull-cracking headache, the aching joints, and the profound fatigue.

The nurse tells him to call an ambulance. The situation is urgent.

I cry. I plead. I can't go back to that emergency room again and I'm determined that my wishes aren't going to be overridden by some disembodied voice that clearly has no experience trying to get healthcare from the godforsaken horror show that passes for the local hospital.

I'm adamant about this. I won't change my mind. Don't even try me.

I don't remember much after that, only fragmentary images with no context to anchor them.

A magnetic attraction to the hospital floor.

The pain of a needle breeching a vein.

Bright lights being shone in my eyes over and over and over again.

I remember all of this from above as I look down at the body on the bed, not quite connecting it to me, and I recall thinking that it no longer matters whether I live or die. Nothing matters anymore.

But then maybe that's just the sort of thing people think when the morphine finally kicks in.

A WEEK LATER

They decide to keep me. Lucky me.

I'm wheeled from the emergency room in the middle of the night and placed in a room alongside a morbidly obese patient who sleeps twenty hours a day and snores loud enough to trigger earthquakes two continents away.

Someone arrives to wake me up at regular intervals.

This really isn't necessary. The non-stop snoring ensures I won't be sleeping anytime soon.

Snort. Snort. Bluster. Snort. It's like lying next to a chainsaw with a faulty motor.

It occurs to me that this is what hospital administrators do to patients who can't take a hint. If a patient keeps coming back to the hospital after doctors have repeatedly dismissed her then they have no choice but to torture her in an effort to make sure that she will never, ever feel the need to come back again.

I feel like a character in a Stephen King novel.

The setting contributes to this feeling. The walls are painted a color that can best be described as drab and the window blinds — which are inexplicably embedded between two panes of glass — are broken, preventing them from being moved from their present position, which is partially raised yet slightly askew. The bed is a ramshackle disaster of technology that I can easily imagine being a cast-off from another, better hospital when it updated its furnishings forty years ago. And just to complete the horror-story effect, the hospital's power goes out several times one day, forcing the back-up generators to kick in and noisily expel stale air from the vents.

Again and again and again.

I half-expect a machete-wielding lunatic to burst into my room. I'm only vaguely surprised when this doesn't happen.

Or maybe it does; it's not like I would remember.

I'm in the hospital for more than a week, but my memory of that time is fragmentary, disjointed, as though someone loaded a random set of slides into a projector and is flashing them on a screen inside my brain without providing any narrative glue.

Slide 1.

Someone is speaking to me — a nurse, I think — but I can't understand what she's saying.

"Source black round fluid next."

"Are you talking to me?"

"Koi freak leaven irritate deer."

"I'm sorry, I don't understand what you're saying."

"Winter serif all?"

"Still not getting it."

"Lewis late episode are ego ant alter window?"

"Look, whatever it is, can you just pretend I gave you the answer you're looking for?"

"Rifle did jelly art kudo?"

"Yes."

"Jungle dime?"

"All right then, no."

"Timeless dark swallow sit table juror dad."

"Screw it. You've got a brain. Whatever it is, just figure it out for yourself."

"Swat whiskey fur."

"Christ."

Slide 2.

A doctor is standing at the foot of my bed, flipping through pages in a chart that's resting on the rolling table where the trays of untouched food usually reside. He's telling me that I could be in the early stages of multiple sclerosis.

Possibly lupus.

Maybe rheumatoid arthritis.

Somehow I get the impression that the choice is mine and I try to consider the pros and cons of each disease, but quickly discover that I don't know enough about any of them to feel confident that I'll choose the one that will be the least destructive in the long run.

The conversation veers in another direction.

I fail to veer with it.

Slide 3.

Pinpoints of phosphorescent light are raining down so thickly I can barely see the wall at the foot of my bed. There are several people in the room — three or four, I think — but they are vague, sketchy, as though they're made of grey fuzz instead of flesh.

Someone asks a question.

Someone else answers.

I say something, but can't understand my own words.

My left hand is tingling in the strangest way and so is my spine. Not all of it, mind you. Just the region from my neck to the bottom of my ribcage.

There's a sudden burst of strangeness at the base of my skull that feels as if someone has shoved an ice pick up into my brain, causing my thoughts to flap around like birds in a hurricane.

Someone touches my shoulder, but I don't know why.

Too much is happening.

I don't know what to focus on.

Slide 4.

A doctor is sitting on a chair at the foot of my bed and I'm trying to decide if it's the same doctor as before. I don't think so, but I'm having trouble distinguishing one person from another so I can't say for sure.

People seem like apparitions.

They're indistinguishable and interchangeable and I can't quite pull them into focus but, on a bright note, I always seem to know which ones the doctors are, something that I'm going to attribute to a survival instinct I didn't know I had.

Anyway, this doctor apparition is telling me that I could have rheumatic fever, West Nile virus or multiple sclerosis. He mentions meningitis, then openly questions whether this could be malaria, and for the first time it occurs to me that infectious diseases are being named alongside autoimmune illnesses.

Can't doctors tell the difference?

I mean, isn't distinguishing between an illness that's caused by infection and one that isn't first-day-of-medical-school sort of stuff? It's clear to me that this doctor is guessing and I'm gazing at him, half-stunned, wondering if he knows that I know all his authoritative banter is designed to cover up a fundamental cluelessness.

Let's hope not.

Nothing positive could come from that.

Slide 5.

The nausea is overwhelming. Soon a nurse arrives with a small bag of fluid and hooks it into my IV. This bag is smaller than the ones that have been hydrating me since I arrived in hospital and I find myself staring stupidly at it as the nurse hooks it up.

Christ, I'm really out of it today.

The fevers usually arrive in the evening and leave by morning. And they're worse every second night.

The fevers. They're the same ones that haunted me months ago and now they've returned, still as predictable as German trains. You could set your watch by them.

Only today you can't. Today they've decided to break with the familiar pattern and burn throughout the day, causing me to stare daftly at a bag of fluid and then at a nurse.

She's shimmering like a mirage above the hot desert sand. I'm riveted.

Until I realize that she's hooking Gravol into my IV in an effort to gain control of the nausea. Bad plan.

Gravol is the one substance on earth that's guaranteed to make me puke, something that I've been fighting valiantly to avoid all morning. And yes, I know that's the opposite of what it's supposed to do, but that doesn't change the fact that that's what happens every single time.

I tell this to the nurse.

She listens and smiles and leaves.

I don't think she likes me much, but then I did just vomit on the cables and cords snaking next to my bed and it's hard to like a person who does something like that.

I do it again.

The puking does nothing to alleviate the nausea, which is so overwhelming that I'm squirming.

An orderly arrives with a wheelchair to take me down to radiology.

I do my best to ignore the nausea.

To pacify it.

To push it down.

I'm wheeled out of the ward, through the emergency room, and into radiology, where x-rays are taken with me standing against a wall like a prisoner about to be shot. I'm so weak I'm not sure my legs will hold me up for as long as they need to — or for as still as they need to — so that the x-rays can be taken.

The nausea is now so powerful that I'm starting to shake. Badly.

I'm a volcano holding down massive amounts of molten lava, not something volcanoes do well.

Still, I do my best — really I do — and I make it through the x-ray. I make it, in fact, as far as the emergency room on my way back to the ward before

I start to spew uncontrollably. Vomit hits the floor and the wall before someone pointlessly drags a trash can over to me and I puke into that.

Repeatedly.

Endlessly.

Honestly, how much vomit can one person generate? It's not like I've eaten much more than toast and Tylenol since arriving at the hospital, so surely my stomach is going to run out of ammunition soon. While I wait for that glorious moment to arrive, I struggle to keep all that wretched slime from getting into my hair, otherwise the stench will surround me like flies on a corpse long after I'm wheeled back to my room. A nurse takes pity on me, brushing my hair away from my face and tying it into a ponytail with a rubber band.

Eventually the vomiting subsides long enough for me to apologize.

I don't know why or to whom, but it's the orderly who shrugs.

"You're not the first person to vomit in an emergency room. You're not even the first person today."

Perspective.

I spend the rest of the day trying to tease the rubber band out of my hair, all the while wondering why I didn't just rip the IV from my arm, preventing the Gravol from running into my system in the first place or, better yet, insist that someone stop the medication for me.

I'm going to blame that on the fever.

It's hard to think straight when a fever turns homicidal.

Slide 6.

A doctor is kneeling at my bedside. He's feeding a needle into a vein that has already had dozens of needles fed into it over the past several days. The pain is alarming and I'm begging him to stop, but he's telling me that I really don't want him to.

My blood holds the key.

Certain tests can only be run if blood is drawn during a febrile state and I'm in that state now, at some ungodly hour of the morning. So the doctor is here and he's drawing my blood and he's being vague about what the test is for.

I squirm and I cringe.

I can't help wondering what a doctor is doing drawing blood from a patient's arm in the middle of the night or, for that matter, at all.

Isn't that someone else's job?

The next morning a lab technician shows up to draw more blood and I start to cry. My arms are in so much pain from all the needles that I beg her not to jab me again. I tell her that a doctor did that in the middle of the night and he seemed confident that the blood he was drawing then would yield the answers he was looking for. Can't we just go with that?

Sadly, it seems that someone put that blood in the fridge, rendering it useless. The technician needs to draw a new sample even though I'm no longer spiking the fever that the doctor seemed to think was so critical to getting accurate test results. I try not to take this in, but inevitably I do, and all I can think is, "Somebody, please, get me out of this hellhole."

✳

Slide 7.

A peculiar feeling is radiating out from the center of my brain.

It's overwhelming, all encompassing, unsurvivable.

I can't stand it and yet I can't get away from it.

Somehow I know, without having to be told, that if I can't shut it down, something devastating is going to happen.

And I can't shut it down.

So the devastating thing happens.

Only I can't remember what it was.

All I know is that I'm staring at a drab wall, in a haze, with a brain that feels like it's been trampled by stampeding elephants and a sense that more time has passed than I'm able to recall. It helps that there's a clock on the wall facing me and its hands are not where they should be, not by a long shot.

What just happened?

And why, for the love of God, do other people pass out when horrific things happen to them while I get to experience the whole bloody thing?

Experience it, yes.

Remember it, no.

My brain knows more than it's telling.

✳

Slide 8.

"What's this?"

"Medication."

"What for?"

"It'll calm you down."

"I don't need calming down."

"It'll make you feel better."

"Not having these attacks will make me feel better."

"It's what we give patients to prevent seizures."

"Twenty minutes ago that might've been useful."

"The doctor wants you to take it."
"The doctor isn't here."
"Can't you just take it?"
"Will it cure me?"
"It'll help you."
"But it won't cure me?"
"It's not that kind of drug."
"Then get me that kind of drug."
"I can only do what I'm told."
"I'm telling you."
"I'll come back later."
"Why bother?"

Slide 9.

It's the middle of the night and a doctor has placed a pillow over my face.

I know what you're thinking, but we haven't drifted that far into Stephen King territory quite yet. The pillow is covering my face because the doctor needs to have the lights on in order to assess the state of things but the light hitting my eyes is light-years beyond painful and I need it off.

Hence the pillow.

The doctor taps my knee with some instrument I can't see and a shiver races up my spine, causing every muscle in my body to abruptly contract. The doctor then taps the other knee and gets the same result. When he taps my ankle, he gets nothing.

He tries the other ankle.

Still nothing.

This sends him back to my knees where his tapping unleashes the same shivers and contracting muscles as before. I don't know why he's doing this and I don't particularly care. He can hit my ankles as many times as he wishes since they're deader than doornails, but he has to stop hitting my knees.

This isn't optional.

A strange feeling erupted somewhere deep inside my brain with the first tap and each successive tap is causing that feeling to swell beyond the point of overwhelming. If he doesn't stop, something awful is going to happen, so I inform him that he's going to get the same reaction every time he hits my knees, making it pointless to continue doing so.

That's the polite version of what I said.

Now imagine that same sentence laced with half a dozen obscenities and delivered at a volume normally reserved for an air raid siren.

You get the picture.

A week passes. I'm still in the hospital with no clear explanation for what's wrong with me. I've heard the names of so many autoimmune and infectious diseases at this point that they just sort of glance off my brain. Multiple sclerosis is the only one that's been mentioned by every doctor, so it's the one I plan on looking up if I ever get out of here.

And yet it doesn't cross the finish line in first place.

In the end, I'm given a clinical diagnosis of relapsing tick fever, put on oral antibiotics, and kept in the hospital for an additional day before finally being released. The reason for the extra day is that spirochetal illnesses — of which relapsing tick fever is one — can sometimes turn homicidal when hit with antibiotics, causing a sudden, temporary amplification of symptoms known as a Jarisch-Herxheimer (or Herx) reaction.

Herx reactions can cause several things to happen.

They can cause blood pressure to initially rise then plummet, rashes to flare, the pulse to race, and fevers to hit the roof before descending into bone-rattling chills. In extreme cases, Herx reactions can be fatal, so the doctor wants to monitor me for twenty-four hours after treatment begins, just in case.

Not that I'm told any of this.

All I'm told is that the antibiotics could make me very sick at first.

Somehow the doctor fails to mention death as a possible side effect of treatment.

It's just as well.

The Herx reaction is a non-event and with that, I'm released from the hospital with a prescription for five days of antibiotics, feeling more or less like something that's just been dragged out from under the wheels of a bus.

Even then I know that this may not be the end of it.

The doctor makes no bones about the diagnosis being a shaky one and warns me that I'll likely need an MRI at a later date to help sort things out. Multiple sclerosis is still on the radar and by now it's come up so often that I'm convinced that when doctors get the opportunity to consider the problem at leisure, that's the ailment that will come up the winner.

Maybe I should've picked rheumatoid arthritis when I had the chance.

PUBLIC HEALTH

I eventually find out that I have Lyme disease from Chris (not his real name). He claims to work for the public health department and when I question him about the disease he's just diagnosed me with, he tells me he's not a doctor.

Maybe he sweeps the floors. It makes sense to me that the guy who sweeps the floors would be the guy that the higher-ups at the health department would volunteer to deliver bad news on their behalf to an unsuspecting stranger.

And Chris definitely has some bad news. He tells me I have Lyme disease.

I tell him he's wrong.

He tells me that he has a copy of my positive tests for Lyme disease on his desk and that makes him right.

This is surely one of the strangest phone calls I've ever received, not least of which because it's the first (and so far only) time I've been diagnosed with a major disease by someone who isn't a doctor. But Chris sounds trustworthy, so what the heck. Even I have to admit that in the space of one sentence, he's given me more actionable information than all of the doctors in the hospital combined.

But Chris is being difficult. It seems this isn't a social call. This is an interrogation.

Where did I travel in the weeks leading up to my hospitalization?

Did I leave the province?

Did I leave the country?

Do I remember a tick bite?

Do I remember a rash?

What treatment did I receive?

What were my symptoms?

Am I sure?

There are so many questions I'm not able to keep up with them all.

I give answers. I hope they're the right ones, but I'm not sure. My brain is scrambled and there's the distinct possibility that I'm distracted. I am, after all, trying to figure out if I've ever heard of Lyme disease before now. I think so. It's named after the town where it was first identified. I don't know why I know that.

And since I can't remember ever hearing of anyone dying from it, I'm sure that I'll be okay.

Or not. Why would the public health department be harassing someone who's just been released from the hospital unless they're certain she's going to croak and they want to extract as much information as they can before she kicks off? Why, in short, would the folks at public health be contacting me at all unless my illness represents a clear and present danger to my community?

Why, indeed.

This isn't the only phone call I receive. Chris phones back a few more times in an effort to clarify the information I've given him. It seems some of the things I've told him don't jibe with what his bosses were expecting to hear. A medical health officer also calls me, as does a doctor from a local clinic, and all of them have one topic on their minds: Lyme disease.

To the best of my knowledge, I'd never met any of these people before the barrage of phone calls. I certainly never gave any of them permission to access any part of my medical files and yet they all have copies of my test results in front of them, compelling them to call me to discuss whatever aspect of those results is most relevant to them. This leads me to wonder just how many people have access to my supposedly private medical information.

Dozens?

Hundreds?

Whether or not I've been stripped of my right to privacy depends on your point of view. The province's Public Health Act allows officials to gather information about me and disseminate it for any number of reasons related to my health or the health of the general public. All because I tested positive for a reportable disease.

Too bad if I don't like it. And I don't.

But that's not what's really irritating me. What's really irritating me is that while my test results are being passed around like cake at a child's birthday party it evidently doesn't occur to anyone whose desk they land on that it might be a good idea for someone to give me basic information about the disease that Chris has put down his broom long enough to diagnose me with.

Giving me information about Lyme disease is clearly not the purpose of any of these calls.

My questions are met with evasions and outright refusals.

No one with or without a medical degree is willing to discuss any part of this disease with me.

To say that I find this puzzling would be to underestimate my ability to generate conflicting emotions.

That I was tested for Lyme disease at all is one step short of a miracle.

The local hospital is staffed by the doctors who practice in the vicinity — most, if not all, of whom are family physicians — and at some point during my hospital stay one of these doctors contacts a specialist in an effort to put a name on the strange illness that's been plaguing me. Although Lyme disease is suggested by that local doctor, the specialist dismisses it.

It seems there is no Lyme disease in the Kootenays.

At least not according to the specialist.

This may come as something of a surprise to the British Columbia Centre for Disease Control (BC CDC), which lists the Kootenays as endemic for the illness. Evidently they failed to consult this specialist before making that determination. If they had, I'm sure he would have set them straight.

At any rate, the specialist counters with another disease he considers more likely: Relapsing tick fever. There are, on average, between two and four cases of relapsing tick fever in the region each year and the distinctive fevers that have been plaguing me convinces the specialist that this is the illness most likely at the bottom of my woes.

Hence the clinical diagnosis of relapsing tick fever.

Since the local doctor had requisitioned the Lyme tests prior to talking to the specialist, he lets them go through, figuring we might as well have the paperwork in my files ruling Lyme out so that we can move forward with the relapsing tick fever diagnosis on firmer ground.

Only the tests don't rule Lyme out.

They rule it in in a major way.

With that, I'm once again placed on oral antibiotics, this time for three weeks. And once again I'm told that I may suffer a Herx reaction and that if things get really bad, I should return to the hospital.

Fat chance. I just escaped that hellhole. I have no intention of going back there anytime soon. I haven't forgotten that doctors spent months telling me there was nothing significantly wrong with me only to concede that there was a problem when the illness inevitably hit a crisis point. I'm convinced that crisis could've and would've been averted if any one of those doctors had taken my concerns seriously. Not one of them did. Until, of course, things had taken a turn for the catastrophic.

Turn to them for help? I don't think so. I only landed in the hospital because some nurse freaked my husband out and he felt he had no choice but to take me there.

So I down the antibiotics like a good, if somewhat indignant patient, hoping against hope that they'll rid me of this vicious monster of a disease once and for all, thereby relieving me of ever having to deal with another doctor again in my life.

And for the first couple of weeks, things seem to be heading in the right direction.

Symptoms start to taper.

For the first time in months, I have the sense that this nightmare might finally be coming to an end. But then, just as the antibiotics are beginning to run out, things take a sudden and dramatic turn for the worse.

And with that, I'm introduced to the awesome wrath of dying Lyme bacteria.

STRUCK BY A METEOR

Lyme disease is caused by *Borrelia burgdorferi* (Bb, for short) and several other closely related species of bacteria. Whatever else Bb may be, it is not a defenseless organism. Researchers believe it manufactures powerful toxins that can result in, among other things, widespread inflammation, brain dysfunction, and hormonal disruption.

These toxins are sequestered within the body of the bacteria while they remain alive.

But nothing lives forever.

When Bb dies off naturally, the bacteria break down and the toxins they once housed are released into the host's body where they, along with the fragmented bits of the bacteria's bodies, amplify symptoms. Thankfully, for most people, Bb is only ever present in small numbers, so symptoms remain a minor albeit persistent problem.

When antibiotics are introduced, however, Bb starts dying in increased numbers and this can cause symptoms to dramatically worsen. If antibiotic treatment commences immediately after initial infection, when Bb is present in limited numbers and in its conventional form, then the resulting Herx reaction can be quite mild, if it shows up at all. It doesn't always. Some people go Herx-free during treatment. Others experience a minimal increase in symptoms.

And then there's me.

Both times I was placed on antibiotics I was warned that a Herx reaction might occur within the first 24 hours and that it could get quite serious. And both times I made it through those first crucial hours with no significant amplification of symptoms, leaving me under the impression that I'd dodged a couple of very large bullets.

What doctors didn't tell me, presumably because they didn't know it themselves, is that Herx reactions in advanced Lyme disease often show up in a weak form 48 to 72 hours after antibiotic therapy commences — not within the first 24 hours typical of acute Lyme — and then return several weeks later, sometimes in a massive form.

It turns out that making it through the first 24 hours of treatment wasn't the cause for celebration I thought it was.

If only I'd known that then.

Not that knowing it would've changed anything. The Herx reaction still would've arrived, it still would've been profound, and I still would've gone down hard. The only real difference is that I would've been prepared for what was going to happen instead of being blindsided. Knocked to my knees by a blow from behind.

If there's one positive thing I can say about Herx reactions, it's that they're illuminating. You see, it doesn't matter if you're told in advance that a Herx reaction has the ability to make you horribly ill because you, me, and everyone else has had the experience of being horribly ill at some point in our lives and have a reference for what that feels like.

But the worst flu of your life can't hold a candle to a Herx reaction. Nothing anyone can say will adequately prepare you for the wrath of dying Lyme bacteria. It's like being struck by a meteor. Only a meteor shows its victim the mercy of an abrupt death.

Lyme is a sadist, which sets a body on fire and leaves it to endlessly burn.

It's morning and my skull is hot enough to crack bone.

Moving my eyes is too painful to contemplate.

The only way I can look from one object to the next is by turning my head like an owl, yet unlike an owl, I have to cover my eyes, otherwise they stutter and blurt. On days when my neck is too stiff to move, I have to turn my whole body.

So I try not to look at things. But that brings little relief. Open or closed, my eyeballs feel as if they've been repeatedly smashed by a hostile elbow.

And then there's the mirror. The last time I looked into it, the whites of my eyes had turned bright pink. So I stopped looking into it.

This is probably just as well since my vision has lost its clarity. I'm not blind, mind you. No, everything is just so blurry that it seems as if someone slathered petroleum jelly over my eyeballs before wrapping them in gauze and firing off flashbulbs in the air all around me.

And then there's my spine. It's vibrating so violently that it pins me to the couch, razor blades shooting out in all directions.

They strike my kidneys.

My tongue.

The back of my eyes.

I'm unable to move and barely able to breathe.

My toes are numb and my hand is sizzling.

My arm is short-circuiting in a dangerous way.

A cold breeze gusts across my left thigh, scales my back, and sweeps over the top of my head where it continues to swirl for hours.

My body temperature blasts through the roof and my blood pressure drops through the floor.

I black out when I try to sit up.

I black out when I roll over.

I black out when lying still.

I black out so many times I dread coming to.

I try to stand up.

I have to.

I need to pee so badly my bladder is bursting, but when I get to my feet everything abruptly turns black and I fall. When I come to, I'm convinced that I'm still falling even though I can feel the floor against the back of my ribs and one of my hips. I must've dislodged the floor when I hit it and together we're falling into some unnamed abyss. I roll onto my back, hoping this will improve the situation, but the sensation that I'm perpetually falling doesn't stop, so I struggle back to my feet where I stagger and sway, hunched over like a prizefighter who's just taken a career-ending blow to the guts.

As I stumble towards the bathroom, the walls liquefy and fold in on themselves like ribbons of warm caramel. Then I collapse like a hot air balloon whose flame has been extinguished.

I get up again.

I still need to pee.

My thoughts are racing. They pour into my brain quicker than I can think them, but they're too unruly to decipher. I can't concentrate on what's going on all around me or even what's happening inside my head.

Everything is spinning so fast.

The floor is slamming up and down beneath my feet like the deck of a ship in hurricane waves. I stagger forward, but I've lost the ability to gauge where body is in relation to the objects around me.

I crash into a wall.

A railing.

A couch.

I'm on my knees.

I reach for a chair and miss, then swing my arm several times like a cat swatting at an invisible Christmas tree ornament. With each swat I inch beyond where my brain is telling me the chair is located until finally I brush it with my fingertips. Later I break a mug trying to put it on a counter that's six inches below where I think it is and jam a finger reaching for a cupboard that's a foot closer than it appears.

But by then I'm too miserable to care.

I'm in the emergency room. I don't know how I got here, but I pretend that I do. That seems like the wisest course of action.

I don't really think anyone here will help me. They never have before. And since I don't believe any planets are currently in a rare alignment, I'm mystified as to why I might have come here. This place is repugnant. It's the one spot on earth I never, ever wanted to be again, and yet here I am.

I feel defeated.

Deflated.

Judging by the electrodes stuck to my chest, my heart misbehaved. That slow-slurring rebel.

Or possibly not.

I recognize the doctor on duty. He once told me he wouldn't investigate more than one symptom at any given time. He must've made the choice himself.

I doubt cardiac arrhythmia is the symptom I would've picked since my heart stopping no longer strikes me as such a bad idea.

Still, it figures he'd be the doctor I'd get. I just can't seem to catch a break these days.

Anyway, my favorite doctor is sitting on the edge of my bed with his fingers wrapped around both of my wrists. Ostensibly he's taking my pulse simultaneously on both arms although I'm not sure I really believe this is his main objective.

He's telling me that he's pulled my hospital records. He's also telling me that those records — the same ones that were used to help other doctors diagnose Lyme disease — indicate to him that my problems, though seemingly medical, are actually psychological.

Records don't lie.

I tell him about the Lyme and about the antibiotics, although I'm sure I must've done this already, but he isn't interested.

Crazy is crazy.

The illness is inconsequential compared to my obvious mental weakness.

He says all this while mispronouncing the name of my disease. Again and again and again. The name of my disease is one syllable long. How could anyone possibly get that wrong?

I don't care.

The whole wrist thing is creeping me out. It occurs to me that the safest course of action is to simply not fight back. I don't have the energy and my left arm has gone numb, so I'm not terribly sure I could fight back if I wanted to.

I only want to go home. So I sit in silence and wait for the doctor to let go of my wrists. And I pretend to believe that he could really be this fascinated by my pulse.

Bruises are fanning out across my thighs.

I'm certain some of them are the result of crashing into objects that weren't located where my brain was telling me they were — positive, in fact — but most of them aren't and I can't even guess at what the underlying cause for those might be.

Each time I look down there are more of them.

Even the ones that I determined might've been the results of collisions seem to be spreading. It's like watching blue-black ink slowly seeping through a paper towel.

The same phenomenon shows up on my upper arms.

A thought occurs to me: Blood vessels are leaking.

I won't let the thought in.

Not all the way.

I can't even imagine why blood vessels would suddenly start to leak.

So I tell myself this isn't happening.

An eternity passes.

Or possibly a second.

Then I start to wonder where else in my body blood vessels might be leaking and my thoughts turn inevitably to my brain.

I pull my skirt down and cover my arms.

Nothing I can't see can possibly hurt me.

I'm willing to bet my life on it.

KNOW THINE ENEMY

Maybe I should take a moment to say a few words about Lyme disease; to give you the background that no one saw fit to give me.

Where do I begin?

How about here: Lyme is the most frequent tick-borne disease in the temperate regions of the world, which include Canada, the United States, Europe, Asia and Japan. That seems like an interesting fact.

Here's another one: Lyme disease is an enigma. The more closely I look it, the less certain I am what it is I'm seeing and yet, like a person watching as a tornado bears down on a small town, I'm powerless to look away. After five long years of studying this disease, I'm not sure I'm getting any closer to the answers I'm seeking. Worse, I'm not sure the so-called experts are either.

What I know for certain is that everything about Lyme disease, right down to its definition, is unstable and open to interpretation. Most references will tell you that the illness is caused by infection with the bacteria Bb, but a growing number of people consider the disease to be caused by a complex of tick-borne pathogens over which Bb, when present, is dominant. Some of those tick-borne pathogens have been identified and given quirky names like *Anaplasma, Babesia, Bartonella, Ehrlichia* and *Mycoplasma*.

Others remain elusive.

And yet while Bb is routinely touted as being the causative agent of Lyme disease, it's just one of several possible — and closely related — bacteria capable of spawning the illness. That group of bacteria includes Bb sensu stricto (meaning "in the strictest sense"), but it also includes *Borrelia garinii, Borrelia afzelii, Borrelia spielmanii, Borrelia bavariensis,* and a handful of others.

Some are so new to us that their scientific names haven't been established yet.

Others are suspected, but not yet proven to exist.

This group of bacteria is collectively known as *Borrelia burgdorferi* sensu lato (meaning "in the broader sense"). It might be interesting to note, however, that depending on where you live in the world, you can contract Lyme disease without ever coming in contact with Bb. Nonetheless, the bacteria get the lion's share of the blame for causing the disease.

However, if you live in Canada, Bb is the only one you're ever likely to hear about.

I'm not sure if that's a good or a bad thing.

It certainly simplifies matters.

I'm just not certain simplifying a complex illness is doing anyone any favors. But then no one is asking me.

Here are a few more neat things I've managed to dig up about Bb: It's a wildly variable species and to date there are known to be at least 300 strains worldwide, of which roughly 100 make their home in North America.

Each of these strains is capable of creating its own unique brand of havoc.

The duration, severity and variety of symptoms a patient develops depends on which strain of Bb they contract (or which species of borrelia they contract, if not Bb sensu stricto), what combination of co-infections come along with it, and how that patient's individual immune system responds to the invading organism(s), if at all.

Not everyone who contracts Bb develops an immune response to it, which means you can have Bb in your system right now and yet have absolutely no symptoms to tell you it's there because your own immune system is failing to alert you.

I'll let you mull that one over for a few minutes before telling you how that can possibly be the case.

A doctor is telling me that I'm peeing blood and I'm trying to look interested.

I've been peeing blood for months now, so this information hardly comes as a surprise.

If the doctor were to suddenly announce that blood is no longer detectable in my urine, I'd find that a newsworthy bit of trivia. An unexpected anomaly.

He clearly isn't saying that. The blood is irritating him. He seems perturbed that it isn't going away on its own.

I feel the same way about Lyme disease, so at least we're both rocking the same emotion even if the causation doesn't quite match up.

Nothing new there, either.

This doctor thinks there's some great mystery about where the blood is coming from. I think that since my left kidney perpetually feels like it's being actively and ruthlessly scrubbed with steel wool, it's likely ground zero for the leak.

The doctor agrees this is a possibility.

A possibility for him is a likelihood for me.

Not exactly a meeting of minds, but close enough.

So, anyway, I'm trying to look captivated by the whole bleeding issue. That's not really why I'm here, so mostly I'm trying not to get sidetracked. No, I'm here because although I was referred to a specialist months ago, an appointment still hasn't been scheduled and I'm growing frustrated. I can't understand how someone with an infectious disease can be left hanging indefinitely. I mean, isn't it the very nature of infectious diseases that you need to move swiftly with them?

Apparently not. Apparently you can take your sweet time with those.

Meningitis, pneumonia, flesh-eating bacteria. What's the worst that could possibly happen if you ignore one of those?

Nothing comes to mind.

But then we aren't talking about one of those, are we? We're talking about Lyme disease and it's in a different class altogether.

A class that can evidently be ignored indefinitely.

This isn't the first time I've complained about not having seen a specialist. I keep on complaining and always I'm told the same thing: The specialist is one very busy dude.

So busy that he can't even schedule an appointment. So busy that five years down the road, he still won't have found the time to schedule an appointment.

I don't think he's trying very hard.

Not that it's a complete mystery why he wouldn't be. It's likely the same reason I'm not a member of his fan club: The specialist I've been referred to is the same one who was consulted while I was in the hospital and who declared that I couldn't possibly have Lyme disease since there is no Lyme in the Kootenays. That my God-like friend was subsequently proven wrong by the medical tests is something that likely doesn't sit well with him. If I were a betting person, I'd put money on never hearing from that specialist. Like most betting people, I think I know a sure thing when I see one.

Still, desperate people do desperate things, so for months I keep on trying to get an appointment with the only specialist within hundreds of miles of my home, all the while wondering when someone is going to have the guts to tell me to my face that I'm out of luck when it comes to receiving information, medical advice, or treatment for my illness.

But then that would be to admit that there's a problem.

And we must never do that.

Now I know you're wondering why your immune system wouldn't respond to an invading pathogen since that's pretty much the definition of what it does, and to answer that I'm going to have to bring up the topic of antigenic variation.

You're going to love this part.

Bb is, if nothing else, a formidable opponent and one that's taken to shape-shifting with a virtuosity normally reserved for the antagonist of a science fiction novel. Like an alien species that can board a spacecraft and suddenly, effortlessly, assume the appearance of the ship's captain, chief medical officer, or engineer in order to fool those whose jobs it is to repel it, when Bb enters the human body it can transform the proteins on its outer surface to mimic those of whatever native body cell it thinks will protect it from attack.

One minute it looks like an invading bacterium.

The next it's indistinguishable from a heart cell, a neural cell, a synovial cell or whatever other kind of cell the immune system will be reluctant to attack.

Bb isn't the only organism that can do this.

Many other species of bacteria, protozoa and fungi — including the pathogens that cause gonorrhea, malaria, and relapsing tick fever — can also vary their antigens, but Bb does so by employing a unique mechanism that scientists are still struggling to get a handle on. However, they have managed to establish that Bb is a surprisingly promiscuous chameleon that rearranges its antigens to a breathtaking extent.

Bb is a born survivor.

It's perpetually ready to alter its structure to meet whatever challenges it encounters from immune response, antibiotics, or anything else that causes a hostile change in its environment. There's no sense looking like a heart cell if looking like a neural cell will confer greater protection at any given moment.

There's a definite logic to the way this bacterium thinks.

A logic I wish my immune system would find a way of unraveling.

Something inside me is peaking and diving with no pilot at the controls to level things out and I'm crying because I'm scared and I'm tired and I'm completely in the dark about what's happening. In the space of an average day, the roller coaster swoops and soars so many times only a savant could keep track of it all.

And I'm not a savant.

I never know what symptom is going to come at me, how hard it's going hit, or how long it's going to stay. All I know is that there's no time to take a breath between rides. Symptoms manifest in clusters, each overlapping with the next. There are never less than a dozen and often there are twenty or thirty in unpredictable combinations, as if there's a roulette wheel hidden somewhere deep inside my body and Lyme is spinning away like a coked-up psychopath.

The one constant is fatigue. It drags me to the floor and holds me there.

Heat blows through me like a desert wind, scorching my left shin, my right eye, my tonsils, my fist.

Lights flicker fast.

The world moves slowly.

I try to think about ponies and ice cream and Paris cafés, but my mind refuses to be distracted by whimsical thoughts. Or, at least, it refuses to be distracted by those whimsical thoughts.

I wonder if all this suffering is karma for the bugs I've squished during my lifetime. I mean, I've squished a lot. Some of them were faultless; others were mosquitoes.

And now all of these insects — every single one of them — have come back to haunt me in the form of spiral bacteria. That's the sort of revelation that could turn me Buddhist in a flash and it irks me because I thought I was supposed to pay for my karmic transgressions in the next lifetime. Isn't that what the books say? If I behave like a saint in this lifetime then I'll reap the rewards in the next, but if I instead behave like an insufferable, bug-zapping harpy then I'll come back as a raccoon or a bat or a disease-ridden nobody.

Karma isn't playing by the rules and that's just not fair. I know. I've read the books.

And yet here I am, stuck in a situation that only karma could've thought up. I've never heard of anyone suffering from the kind of chaos I'm suffering from and I don't know where to turn for help. There's no point in going to an emergency room unless I'm willing to whittle down my complaints to just one.

I've been warned.

But I don't know which symptom to pick since a single symptom isn't my problem and pulling one out of the present cacophony is unlikely to get at the heart of the problem, or maybe it will, if I pick the right symptom, but no one is going to help me choose and it strikes me that trying to pluck a snowflake from an avalanche is a dangerous waste of time.

Bb can rearrange its antigens so dynamically because it contains more DNA replicons than any other known bacteria and it's those replicons that allow it to spontaneously and continuously switch around the components of its outer surface so that it can appear to be something it isn't.

Why does that matter?

It matters because these outer surface proteins are what identify Bb (or any other invader) to the immune system, so strategically altering these proteins allows the invading bacterium to avoid detection by the immune cells that are designed to hunt it down. Confused, these protector cells don't know what to attack and, like the spaceship's crew that finds itself face-to-face with someone who may or may not be their captain, they must decide whether to attack based on little more than gut instinct.

Fine in a comic book. Not so fine in a human body.

It's an ingenious defense, really. Even I have to admit that. It's also enormously inconvenient if you happen to be the person the bacterium is infecting, since the net result is what appears to be the body's equivalent of a mutiny: an autoimmune attack. This results in Lyme patients like me being told we may be suffering from any one of an impressive number of incurable autoimmune illnesses.

Lupus erythematosus.

No, wait.

Multiple sclerosis.

No, no. Give me a minute here.

Rheumatoid arthritis.

That's it.

Is that it?

Although the immune system is doing its best to fulfill its primary function, it finds itself caught in a distressing situation where the enemy can be anything, anywhere, and probably is.

Someone looking at the situation without knowing all of the facts might think that a mutiny is underway when the opposite is true; the crew members are trying valiantly to do the right thing in the face of an opponent they cannot identify, using tactics they don't understand, and who will ultimately take control of the vessel unless they does something to stop it.

So the crew guesses.

And sometimes it guesses wrong.

Then your hand starts to tingle or your joints start to ache or your heart skips a beat.

Possibly two.

And all because of measures your immune system is taking to defeat an opponent it can sense, but cannot see.

There are days when I wish my immune system would just give up.

Most days, in fact.

I can see the damage it's doing as it tries to defend me against this diabolical invader.

I just can't see the benefits.

If my immune system is under the impression that it's on its way to a glorious victory, I'm afraid I'm going to have to disagree with it there.

What it's doing is destroying me.

One cell at a time.

And regardless of whether or not that's its intent, that's the only area in which it's racking up successes.

And it's racking them up to Olympic extremes.

I break down and go to the hospital.

Even I knew I was going to do that.

The breaking point is the devastating pain in my left kidney. It feels like someone dipped it in battery acid then shoved it back in my body without bothering to use a scalpel. Or anesthetic. Or closing the wound when they were done.

By the time I get to the hospital the pain has gone so far off the top of the scale it no longer registers as pain. It now registers as some kind of turbulent vertigo-nausea hybrid and this leads to some interesting problems.

The main problem is that the doctor doesn't believe I'm in any pain. He calls me a liar to my face.

The second problem is that he wants to give me Gravol for the nausea and I consider it, really I do, but ultimately I don't see how puking my guts out is going to improve the situation, so I tell him what happens when I take Gravol, thinking, rather naively, that we can move on from there to something a little more useful.

The doctor, however, tells me that what I'm saying is impossible.

I respond by reciting the dictionary definition of impossible and contrast it to an adverse reaction to medication. I mean, it's clear that this doctor doesn't quite grasp that impossible is fairly universally defined as something that isn't possible, so I do my duty as a defender of the English language by informing him of this.

He goes ballistic and starts to shout.

I return fire.

The visit goes down in a hail of verbal bullets and I storm out of the ER like John Wayne striding away from a battlefield. Yeah, right. I look more like Gumby stumbling out of a bar after a drinking spree, but the John Wayne imagery helps me to preserve some sense of dignity, so that's the imagery I'm determined to embrace. Regardless of which screen icon I look more like, I leave in a huff, and since I'm not entirely certain where solid objects are located in relation to my body, I find them by colliding with them, and I'm limping because moving my left leg is making the nausea significantly worse. It's also threatening to reignite the cataclysmic kidney pain and I absolutely do not want that reignited. So I limp and I whimper and I aim for the car.

My husband, who watched in dismay as this whole thing went down, returns to the emergency room and tries to reason with the doctor, coming back a few minutes later with a prescription for anti-nausea medication that will never be filled. Somehow this is supposed to be a peace offering. I'm not entirely certain I understand how.

Instead I've turned my attention to hoping that whatever is wrong with my kidney will magically go away on its own, but hope isn't enough to erase the knowledge that I'm pretty cursed in the luck department these days, so I cry all the way home from the hospital.

And I'm pondering how I'm going to dull the pain engulfing my kidney. I consider taking the long, lonely drive to that other, better hospital almost two hours up the road, but I'm not at all sure I'm physically capable of making it that far.

I can't make it that far.

I'm pretty much screwed.

It's not that I don't have any painkillers. I have them all right, but instead of reducing the kidney pain — which is the reason they were given to me in the first place — they increase it exponentially and cause me to pee blood. Or, I should say, they cause me to pee more blood than I normally do. This blood I can see. It's not just something that shows up on a urine test and irritates a doctor who is hoping against hope that clicking his heels together will make it go away.

Anyway, I'm considering taking those painkillers, not because I think they'll dull the pain, but because I'm hoping they'll succeed in blowing out my left kidney much like a tire hitting a mat of spikes. It's either that or I'm going to have to break a bottle and gouge that kidney out myself.

Anything would be less painful than this.

PEEKING BENEATH THE MASK

So who is this invader that wears the masks of the innocent to perpetrate crimes against its host?

I'm far from the first person to ask this question and in 1997 researchers succeeded in mapping Bb's genome — the genetic material that comprises the bacterium — in a quest to better understand its oddly destructive behavior. In doing so, they discovered that Bb contains just shy of 1,300 genes, which together control everything from its digestive and reproductive functions to its ability to mutate to address any hostile changes in its environment.

Dozens of these genes control proteins whose biological functions remain unknown.

What is known is that they've only ever been seen in other spirochetes. (I'll get to what a spirochete is in a minute. Be patient. I need to dazzle you a little first.)

Bb also has more plasmids (bundles of DNA) than any bacterium recorded to date. Bb is indeed one complex little creature.

It's this genetic material that allows Bb to tinker with its outer surface proteins swiftly and frequently, coming up with sequences that can be unique on each individual Bb bacterium in my body and different from anything that exists in the infecting tick.

Now, Bb isn't the only organism that can perform these genetic gymnastics.

The organisms that cause relapsing tick fever and syphilis employ much the same strategy and yet how exactly they accomplish it remains largely unknown.

What is known is why: survival.

By the time Bb is injected into a human body, it has already lived in at least one other mammal as well as the ticks that transported it from one mammal to the next. In order to survive in these disparate hosts, Bb had to learn how to successfully evade the attacks of sophisticated and diverse immune systems and that's no mean feat.

Most bacteria can only dream of doing that.

In order to accomplish this, Bb has evolved over thousands of years so that it can rapidly adapt to the hostile environments present in any number of hosts determined to use anything and everything in their arsenals to annihilate it. The survival mechanisms that work best in a tick's gut are unlikely to be successful when Bb is injected into a mouse, a deer or me. Survival in these varied conditions requires superlative adaptability.

And Bb has proven itself to be more than up to the challenge.

Rashes are swarming my body. They kaleidoscope within borders of their own creation and when I examine the one spanning my stomach, it looks very much like someone pressed a swatch of paisley fabric against my skin, then pulled it away, leaving a furious collection of red swirls in its wake. Last week there was a similar rash across my back, and yesterday the rashes on my calves bore an uncanny resemblance to scarlet scatter-shot.

The patterns revolve and evolve as the hours go by and watching them is like watching the rise and fall of entire civilizations, time-lapsed to span hours instead of centuries. Sometimes a rash will burble with tiny blisters like some biblical plague or sprout a random collection of pimples that spread out across the redness like tiny personalized constellations.

Despite the constantly evolving details, these rashes subscribe to a fundamental organizing principle: They are always bilateral. If there's a rash on my right thigh, there will invariably be a matching one on my left. The same is true when they show up on my forearms, hands, or the tops of my feet. When they appear like exotic butterflies across my face, stomach or back, they are equally balanced between left and right.

My skin is a canvas under the brush of an artist I cannot see. And it's a gentle artist. I have to see these rashes to know they exist because I can't feel them. I can press on them, blow hurricanes across them, even run my tongue over their strange patterns and they feel no different than the unaffected skin just inches away.

Sight is the only sense that registers them.

But if I step into the sun, even for a moment, all that changes.

These benign rashes are joined by another rash, this one faint and pink and furious. It extends from the top of my head to the bottom of my feet and burns like a tire fire that nothing on heaven or earth can extinguish.

Ask me how I know.

Bb belongs to a class of bacteria known as spirochetes. This class is named for the notable characteristic that its members all possess: They look like spirals. By far the best known of these spiral bacteria is *Treponema pallidum,* the bacterium that causes syphilis.

But Bb's classification as a spirochete can be a bit misleading.

Bb has no close relatives amongst the spiral bacteria it's classified with except for other borrelia species. Although *Treponema* bacteria are the closest non-borrelia species, the organisms share less than 50 percent of their genetic material, making them distant relations indeed.

Not the sort that shows up at family reunions. More the sort that exist as a name on some distant branch of the family tree.

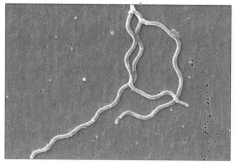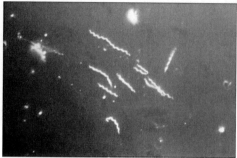

Borrelia burgdorferi

Countless centuries of independent evolution have made it so that *Treponema* and *Borrelia* don't have a whole lot in common these days, at least not as far as genetic structure is concerned. But both are shaped like spirals. Well, sort of.

I should probably point out that although Bb is classed as a spiral bacterium, it doesn't look a whole lot like a spring. If you look at a microscopic photograph, you'll discover that Bb looks less like a coil and more like a fragment of yarn that's been unraveled from a tightly woven sweater.

These photographs can be hard to come by.

Bb has the distinction of being both the longest and skinniest of all known borrelia species and it's this skinniness that makes it hard to see Bb under a microscope unless special lighting or stains are used.

And you've got to see it before you can photograph it.

Still no specialist.

Still peeing blood.

Medical file as thick as a phone book. I had one doctor for thirty-four years and his entire file on me consisted of a few pages. In the space of six months, my file is now hefty enough to break a foot if dropped.

Or thrown. I'm contemplating throwing it now because a doctor has said something to me and I'm wondering how to react. What he has said, essentially, is that judging by the number of times I've shown up at the emergency room and doctor's offices in the past few months, I must really be craving the attention.

I wonder how many cancer patients are told the same thing?

Or patients with diabetes.

I'm guessing any doctor who said that to a patient with either of those diseases would be reprimanded in a hurry.

But my dear friend Lyme is in a class all of its own. Which puts me in a class all of my own. A class that allows doctors to vent their frustrations on its sufferers with no realistic fear of censure.

Bb has an interesting structure that includes a double cell wall composed of an inner membrane and an outer wall that houses up to a dozen whip-like flagella. These flagella are what enable Bb to twizzle around in the spaces between body cells like tiny self-powering drill bits.

Interesting though that is to visualize, let's forget the flagella for a minute.

It's the outer wall that interests us here.

That cell wall is covered in slimy goop, which can present a real challenge to any white blood cell trying to glom onto it. These immune cells find it difficult to envelop such a goopy organism and those that succeed have trouble digesting it, so it's not at all unusual for Bb to pop out of these cells to continue traveling through your body cloaked in the DNA of the cells that tried to swallow it.

That's good news for Bb.

Not such good news for the body under siege, since that cloak is now identifying Bb to the immune system as a native body cell and the immune system is loath to attack one of those.

Most of the time, anyway.

Didn't I used to sleep all the time?

My hibernation has drawn to a close. Now I'm awake twenty hours a day for days, even weeks, on end. During the daytime I'm stupid and clumsy and so exhausted that I wonder where I'll find the energy to move or even breathe. On those rare occasions when I do manage to drop off, I fail to dream. Instead, I wake after an hour or two, exhausted, and meander through another day.

Technically I'm awake, but I have no more life in me than a crash test dummy.

If you were to put me in a car and ram it into a wall, I doubt I'd even notice.

And yet when midnight rears its ugly head, I'll be so wired that I'll fidget and tussle with the sheets. That's why tonight, as I hover in that twilight of consciousness when the waking mind normally gives way to dreams, I pray for carbon monoxide to filter into my bedroom, a gift from an angel or an ancestor or one of the lesser gods.

Instead numbness sweeps through my body, leaving me unable to move, not even to scream, and yet I hear a persistent low moan. It takes me a few seconds to realize that the moaning is coming from me and then a few more before I determine there's nothing I can do to stop it.

I'm trapped between two worlds, granted privileges in neither, and there's no telling how long I remain here. Time doesn't exist in this space. It's just me and eternity and that infernal moaning.

I wish I could snap my fingers and break the spell. I wish I could move my fingers to snap them. I wish a lot of things.

Sometimes at night when sleep refuses to come, I lie flat on my stomach and listen to the sounds in my neck. They are strange sounds, like those a rowboat makes as it grinds lazily against a wooden dock. I imagine tendons winding around bone, cartilage dissolving then reforming like slow-cooling rubber, veins twizzling like worms on hot cement. What's really happening during these moments is a mystery and one I haven't solved by combing through books or seeking the opinion of a qualified expert.

There are no experts, not when it comes to Lyme disease.

So in the darkness I listen to my body with the curiosity of an explorer tracking down the source of whispers that echo from the mouth of some desolate cave. I've become a voyeur who spies on her own body, a body that has become as foreign and as mysterious as the creatures that collect around deep ocean vents.

And what do I listen for?

A low growl at the base of my skull, an unraveling that I feel as much as hear. This unraveling releases the tension from my tongue and for a few fleeting seconds in the dark and the silence of the pre-dawn hours, it feels as though it once again fits comfortably in my mouth.

The effect is ephemeral.

By the time the dull morning light leaks into my bedroom, my tongue is once again thick, slow, weighed down from behind by an anchor so heavy it takes everything I've got to keep it from retreating down my throat.

I remember a time when I could lie on my back and peacefully dream. Now I lie on my stomach for fear that I'll swallow my tongue or choke on the saliva that leaks from my lips now that I've lost the ability to swallow.

Peace is nowhere to be found, not when I'm fighting off the fevers and the shaking and the brilliant white light that has replaced the darkness whenever I close my eyes.

It's hard to sleep when the light in your head never shuts off.

Not impossible, of course.

Anyone who has ever fallen asleep on a bright summer afternoon will testify that sleep can overtake you with the lights fully ablaze. I may have fallen asleep myself on a beach in those halcyon days before a gasp of sunlight became all it would take to ignite my skin and force me into the shadows like an oversized fungus.

An oversized fungus is exactly what I feel like most days.

Years ago, when I was young and darkness was so easy to come by, I used to believe that monsters lay hidden within its folds, waiting for me to fall asleep so that they could sneak out of the shadows and eat my brain.

I know better now.

Those brain-eating monsters are drawn to the light that they themselves switch on and they aren't the size of giants, as I'd once imagined, but are so small they're invisible to the human eye and even to microscopes unless stained with chemical dyes or subjected to special lighting.

But I was right about the hiding.

The bacterium that causes Lyme disease hides inside my body's own cells and in impenetrable cysts of its own design. It even cloaks itself in lymphocytes, a type of white blood cell that manufactures the antibodies that are supposed to hunt down the bacterium so that my immune system can kill it. Only the thing my immune system is supposed to be killing is hiding inside one of its own agents.

Brilliant.

It's like trying to do battle with trained assassins.

These microscopic terrorists are designed to survive everything God and man have invented to bring them down. They dodge antibiotics and fake out my immune system so perfectly that it doesn't know what to attack, so it ends up attacking me. And they lie in ambush, not moving, not making a sound, until all signs point to them having vacated the premises.

Then they come out fighting.

Those battles have left glitches in my nervous system that will never go away, but they've also altered my dreams.

My dreams no longer carry messages from my subconscious.

They don't speak to me in images borrowed from television or drawn from the waters of some deep archetypal well. Nor do they speak to me in metaphors that are sometimes obvious, sometimes obscure; brain puzzles that my mind can endlessly untwist in an attempt to decode the mysteries of life or discover the answer to a problem that's been haunting me for days.

My dreams no longer speak to me in the baffling language of the subconscious.

They no longer speak to me at all.

On those days when mania sweeps through me like a toxic effluent, I will tell you with the intensity of a quasar fighting against its own destruction that I miss my old life; a life where pain was transient, energy seemed boundless, and darkness came with a guarantee.

But that isn't really true.

What I miss are my dreams.

They were complicated and elusive.

They were the products of an endlessly expressive psyche that never seemed to tire in its need to communicate.

Now my dreams speak to me of nothing.

They've abandoned me in the glare of a blinding white light that I stare at from dusk until dawn, waiting for something, anything, to finally release me.

Nothing ever does.

Among the fascinating bits of trivia that surround Bb is the fact that it was originally classified as a protozoan (a single-celled microscopic organism) until it was reclassified as a bacterium (a single-celled organism without a nucleus or organelles).

This is where things get interesting.

Bb is single-celled and doesn't possess a formal nucleus, which is certainly in line with its current classification, but Bb does possess organelles, something that, strictly speaking, bacteria aren't supposed to have, and it has a linear chromosome instead of the circular kind more typical of bacteria.

These things make it a bit of an in-betweener.

Not quite a bacterium.

Not quite a protozoan.

You need a shoehorn to force it into either category and so its leap from one classification to the other — something that's extremely rare — can be explained by it not truly belonging to either, and since there's no place else to stick it, it gets rammed rather awkwardly into an existing category in spite of its anomalies.

But forget all that.

What's really important here — assuming you're the one who is trying to outwit a creature that possesses better survival skills than you do — is that Bb requires fats, sugars and other substances for its survival and yet has evolved to the point where it's incapable of manufacturing these things itself, so it needs to get them from you, me or any other creature it happens to be inhabiting.

So let's call Bb what it truly is: A parasite.

Without a host from which it can siphon the nutrients it needs to sustain its own life, Bb will surely die.

That makes things simple then.

Bb needs me.

But I don't need it.

Let's just hope the bacterium has brains enough to figure that out before it succeeds in stopping my heart.

Morning.

My skull has taken a turn for the atomic.

There's nothing that can touch this kind of pain — at least nothing I have a prescription for — and going to the emergency room means dealing with a doctor, which invariably means groveling and humiliation.

And I won't grovel, not anymore.

I consider my options and discover that I don't have any.

The vertebrae in my neck are fused so tightly that bending my neck forward or moving my eyes in any direction are painful impossibilities. I can't sit up without blacking out and even if by some miracle I could vault myself up onto my feet, vertigo will take me down faster than gravity can carry me.

I fall at the speed of light.

And falling would be bad, although, come to think of it, it's hard to imagine any resulting injury could possibly compete with the intense pressure at the base of my skull.

It's unbearable.

All I can do is scream and flail and hope against hope that the pressure will achieve its goal of crushing my brain stem. And while I'm doing all this hoping, I lie on my side with my head carefully positioned on my saliva-stained pillow imagining that my screams are being swallowed by a vacuum, a black hole, a vast space at the end of time.

Not that any of this helps.

TEXAS ON A WARM SPRING MORNING

Insects are clambering over my calves.

They're conducting frantic searches for whatever it is these creatures search for in the middle of the night.

I have no idea what that might be.

If they were alive, I'd say food.

But they aren't alive.

They're not even dead.

I switch on the lamp and throw back the covers, but see nothing.

This has been going on for hours, weeks, months.

These phantom insects show up in the middle of the night and although I can feel them scuttling across my legs like panicked soldiers storming a beachhead, I haven't once seen them, not even the silhouettes of their bodies as they scramble to and fro under the cover of my skin.

I try a few more times to glimpse them, then take a different tack, distracting myself by making up names for these phantoms. There must be dozens of them, ranging in size from millipedes to ground beetles, and all of them now bear the names of cars.

Edsel.

Studebaker.

Dodge.

Toyota.

DeLorean.

I lose interest in the name game and instead start imagining what a millipede might look like under my skin.

Or a ground beetle.

Or nothing at all.

I wonder what my skin would look like if it encased nothing.

No bones or blood or cartilage.

Not even air.

My skin lying on the ground like a rejected condom.

Now there's a thought.

Maybe it's time to take my brain in a different direction.

Bb isn't particularly fond of blood. That's a surprising thing to learn when you consider that the bacteria got into my body through the bite of an infected tick, which just happened to be taking a leisurely drink of, you guessed it, my blood.

But blood is fluid, watery. For an adept swimmer it's a dream come true.

But Bb isn't an adept swimmer. It's more of a twizzler and blood is a tricky substance to twizzle around in, so once the bacterium was launched into my bloodstream, it set off in search of a viscous material that would allow it to move around more easily.

That viscous material is collagen. It comprises roughly 30 percent of all the protein in our bodies. It's found in our muscles, tendons, ligaments, cartilage, heart, organs, skin, joints, bones, teeth, eyes, mucous membranes, blood vessels and, well, you get the picture. The stuff is literally everywhere, and once Bb discovers it, it bids farewell to the bloodstream and starts twizzling though anything and everything containing collagen.

And that's pretty much anything and everything.

One of the neat things about Bb's genetic structure is that a surprising six percent of it is devoted to movement, so it's no real surprise that Bb is very good at getting where it's going quickly and efficiently.

It can move forwards or backwards at will.

It can move in one direction for a prolonged period of time or repeatedly switch directions if that's the best way to get where it wants to be. When it encounters a barrier, it can even spin like a drill bit and bore though tissue. Bb is so agile, in fact, that there are recorded cases of it twizzling from the site of initial infection to the central nervous system in a matter of hours.

So much for the blood-brain barrier. It's supposed to guard against this sort of thing, preventing foreign invaders, including Bb, from making their way out of my blood stream and into my brain.

That's the whole point.

Did it do that? Did it?

Evidently it didn't get the memo.

Granted the blood-brain barrier is semi-permeable, not bulletproof, kind of like how the wall separating Mexico from the United States is semi-permeable. So I sit here, as secure as Texas on a warm spring morning, contemplating the acrobatic bacteria performing circus stunts in my brain while my body's security forces run around in circles, not entirely certain what to do about the situation, and just generally being incompetent.

And yet you can't fire your own immune system.

Am I the only one who thinks that's unfair?

The fever strikes from nowhere and within minutes it seems to me that it's become the single leading cause of global warming, well ahead of smoke stacks and farting cows. My spine is sweating and the sheets are unbearably humid. I'm paralyzed by a violent, jerky shaking that's getting more urgent the higher my temperature rises.

My body is raging. It's scorching the air. The sky. The low-hanging moon.

The fevers and shaking go on for most of the night and somewhere around dawn it occurs to me just how lonely I am. I push the thought away, but another, more dangerous thought replaces it: If only I can string together five symptom-free minutes, I might actually survive.

But I can't. And I can't take much more of this unrelenting torture.

The only positive here is that I'm afraid to die. If I weren't, I would've ended all of this long ago. I have the power to do that. It may be the only power I have left.

I'd say something deeply philosophical here — something about the meaning of life or the inevitability of death — but I have an urgent concern that philosophy can't address. Specifically, I'm stuck on my stomach in much the same way that turtles get stuck on their backs. Well, actually, it's not quite the same, since turtles can flail their limbs in endlessly creative ways until they succeed in flipping themselves over. No matter how hard I try, I can't make my legs move and I'm not entirely sure why. My legs are ignoring the commands my brain is sending them.

My legs have gone rogue.

Enough. I grab the edge of the bed and twist my upper body so that my shoulders lie flat against the mattress. Torque alone causes my hips to follow suit and at about the halfway point, my legs agree once again to be under my brain's command.

In truth, this whole exercise has been pointless since there's no particular reason I need to move my legs. I just need to know that I can.

The amount of Lyme bacteria present in the human body at any given time is surprisingly low considering the degree of distress the disease can cause, and since my shape-shifting friend is so good at what it does, the human body — that means your body — doesn't necessarily even realize it's been invaded.

That's because Bb often evokes little in the way of an immune response.

It's estimated that up to 20 percent of people infected with Bb never produce any antibodies to the infection.

Talk about stealth.

This lack of immune response means that Bb can be present in your body right now and you don't even know it because you're either symptom free or you're experiencing such minor symptoms that you can easily ignore them. After all, it isn't unusual for joints to ache or fatigue to arise on occasion. Neither of these things necessarily means you have Lyme disease. They could mean that you have teenagers, a nasty boss, or a penchant for overdoing it while plucking dandelions from your lawn.

But then one day something happens.

Maybe you have minor surgery.

A dental procedure.

A car accident.

Possibly you catch your spouse cheating.

Fail to catch your accountant plundering your bank accounts.

Find yourself taking steroids in an attempt to rid yourself of a rash that's been haunting you for weeks.

It doesn't really matter what the stressor is, what matters is that it arrives, and it starts taxing your immune system, lowering it just enough for Bb to gain the upper hand. Then something starts to go terribly, mysteriously wrong with your body.

It can be absolutely anything.

That's the beautiful thing about Lyme disease. It can produce any possible symptom in all possible systems.

These symptoms don't even have to make sense.

It's more typical of Lyme if they don't.

And if you live in Canada, you'll likely find yourself at the mercy of a doctor who has no idea what the symptoms of Lyme disease might be — or worse — who decides he or she does know what they are based on inadequate, outdated or bizarrely misinterpreted information.

Lyme disease won't even be suspected.

But multiple sclerosis might be. Or colitis, or Parkinson's disease, or Meniere's syndrome. Possibly even menopause or some vaguely defined virus.

That's the day your life will change forever.

Your disease may ultimately get a name, true enough; it just may not be the right one and chances are neither you nor your doctor will twig to that fact.

And no one will ever be held accountable for the mistake.

That's the beauty of our medical system.

A doctor can make a mistake and as long as it is considered to be a reasonable one — like telling someone with Lyme disease that they have multiple sclerosis — then no crime has been committed. After all, any of that doctor's colleagues could have made that same error and the truth is, with our doctors' current level of knowledge regarding Lyme disease, it's practically guaranteed they will.

Here's what really boils my blood: I was diagnosed with Lyme disease months ago and not one doctor has been ready, willing, or able to tell me anything about the disease. Nothing. Nada. Zip.

It's not like I haven't asked. I've asked every doctor unfortunate enough to wander into my sights to tell me what's happening to me, where these awful symptoms are coming from, and why I don't appear to be cured, when I took the antibiotics I was given like the good little patient I can sometimes be. I keep asking these questions and I keep getting nowhere.

It's not like any of these doctors have come straight out and admitted that they don't know a single useful thing about Lyme disease. No, they never say that. They dodge. They parry. They deflect. They do anything and everything they can think of to get me out of their faces as quickly as they can without actually having to admit that they don't know anything about Lyme disease other than what they've just looked up in a database. If they even bothered to do that.

I'll give one doctor credit. He actually starts to babble about some rather nefarious-sounding syndrome that Lyme disease patients can sometimes experience after successful treatment for the disease, a syndrome that can cause symptoms to continue to manifest even though the bacteria itself has been killed. When I ask what the features of that syndrome are, he fumbles, failing to name a single one.

How did I know that would be the case?

IMPROPER CHANNELS

Bb can do more than alter its outer surface proteins in an effort to survive the attacks of a riled-up immune system. When the bacterium senses a hostile change in its environment, it can miraculously switch from a vulnerable twizzle of microscopic yarn to a boulder-shaped cyst, and it can make this switch in less than an hour.

It doesn't matter whether the hostile change is due to immune response, nutrient starvation, increased body temperatures, a dramatic change in pH, or an influx of antibiotics — all things that normally strike fear into the hearts of bacteria. Once Bb senses a change, any change, that might put its existence in peril, it makes the transformation.

And it can be quite the challenge to get at Bb while it remains in these cysts.

The immune system boggles.

So do the antibiotics traditionally used to treat Lyme disease.

A class of antibiotics that's come to be known as "cyst-busters" must be implemented if there's to be any chance of gaining an upper hand against these cysts, but even those are only marginally successful, leaving sufferers with months or years of treatment ahead of them with no guarantee of a cure at the end of it all.

It's a good time for Lyme sufferers to pray.

It's a good time for Lyme bacteria to prey.

Bb can remain encysted for extended periods of time. How long is a matter of some debate, but researchers have shown that it can remain encysted for up to ten months and there's reason to believe it can hold course for much longer, possibly even decades.

Bb bides its time.

When it senses the coast is clear, it springs from these cysts, once again transforming into the spiral form it uses to twizzle through collagen on its way to colonizing new areas of the body and brain.

Maybe "springs" isn't quite the right word.

Although the process can begin almost immediately, it can take up to six weeks to complete, but the fact that it can do it at all is pretty awesome.

Now, Bb twizzling through its host's body may seem like a bad thing, but it's also rather fortuitous since that twizzling spiral is the one form Bb takes that's readily accessible to antibiotics and immune attacks, assuming, of course, that your immune system recognizes Bb for what it is and doesn't think it's one of the friendly cells it's not supposed to be attacking.

While ensconced in these protective cysts, Lyme is doing so much more than hiding. It's also producing a whole new generation of spirochetes and, when the surrounding environment is once again to its liking, the spirochete that originally formed the cyst breaks out, along with all of its progeny, and together they twizzle through the body and brain.

And although Bb has no compunction about changing into cysts at the drop of a hat, a certain percentage of the bacteria are always encysted, even under ideal conditions. There are even instances when Bb is present only in its survival forms (no spirals), greatly increasing the chances that at least one of the invaders will survive anything and everything that's thrown at it.

And one survivor is all it takes to start a whole new generation.

I tried to do things the right way. I tried to go through proper channels to get help. But proper channels have gotten me nowhere. Worse. Every contact with the healthcare system diminishes me.

Leaves me one step closer to death. That can't be right. It certainly isn't just. My brain is blowing springs like some B-movie robot.

So I contact a Lyme advocacy group and I'm given the number of a doctor who knows something about this disease. But there's a catch. I'll have to travel hundreds of kilometers to get to him.

I'm in no condition to even sit up for extended periods, so hundreds of kilometers might as well be where the moon is located.

But I'm desperate and grasping, so I take the trip, knowing that my spine will shoot daggers. My brain will spin like a top. The base of my skull will feel as if someone rammed a tennis ball through it.

And I make the trip in the full knowledge that the painkillers haven't yet been invented that can address the kind of pain that's about to rip through my body.

When Bb enters the central nervous system (CNS) — a process that usually takes several days or even weeks, but which in some cases can take as little as a few hours — it behaves differently than it does when it's twizzling around in the body. Within twenty-four hours of gaining entry to the CNS, Bb begins to encyst and, thanks to the miracle of antigenic variation, soon bears little resemblance to the bacteria found elsewhere in the body.

You can thank the blood-brain barrier for that one.

It may not keep Bb out of the brain, but it does create enough of a barrier that the bacteria in the CNS evolve separately from the bacteria in the rest of the body, essentially creating two completely different strains inside one person. If you were to somehow manage to extract the bacteria from the body or brain (or both) of a Lyme sufferer and compare it to the strain of Bb found in the tick that originally caused the infection, chances are excellent that they wouldn't match.

Lyme sufferers breed strains of bacteria within their bodies that are optimized for the unique conditions found inside each of them and since each individual bacterium can evolve separately from every other bacterium inside that host, depending on what alterations they feel are necessary to increase their chances of survival, the mind boggles at just how many permutations of a single organism could potentially be found inside a single person.

Too many.

While Bb bacteria are ensconced in the CNS, they can cause dysfunction in any of the cells they infest. They can also cause an increase in a substance that breaks down myelin sheaths (the substance that encases nerves in much the same way that plastic insulation encases electrical wires). When these sheaths start to break down, patients exhibit symptoms that look very much like those seen in multiple sclerosis (MS): dizziness, poor balance and co-ordination, cognitive impairment, depression, bipolar disorder, impaired speech, impaired swallowing, fatigue, weakness, difficulty walking, hormonal instability, electric shocks down the spine, blurred vision, tremors, muscle spasms, tingling sensations, heat intolerance, pain, pain, pain and more pain.

The good news is that in spite of the chaos they provoke, there are never very many spirochetes in the CNS at any given time. If the disease is promptly diagnosed and treated with antibiotics that are capable of entering the brain in large enough doses to kill the bacteria, there's a reasonable chance that the body will be able to repair the myelin sheaths without leaving behind the lesions that cause the permanent disabilities seen in MS.

That's a big if.

Canada has the distinction of having one of the highest rates of MS in the world and one of the lowest rates of confirmed Lyme disease infections of any northern temperate region, this despite sharing a border with American states known to have staggering numbers of Lyme infections. This begs the obvious question: How many Canadians are being told that they have MS when what they really have is Lyme disease?

No one currently knows the answer to that question.

Suffice to say that many people in this country who turned out to be suffering from advanced Lyme disease were initially told they were suffering from MS. And many people who have been diagnosed with MS have never been adequately investigated for Lyme, something that may ultimately turn out to be a tragic oversight.

I don't regret traveling to see the only doctor willing to help me, although I have to confess that it's an odd experience sitting in his office. I'm dizzy and I'm disorientated and I'm distracting myself from the pain locking up my joints by concentrating on the more familiar pain twisting through my left kidney.

The fatigue is suffocating.

My heart is skipping like a badly scratched record.

Whenever the doctor asks me a question, I repeat his words into my brain to help them gain traction so that I can tease an answer out of the few synapses still firing. I'm so weak I'm sure I'm going to faint or hyperventilate or astral project, so when the doctor tells me I have Lyme disease, I rest my forehead on his desk and tell him that I already know that. Then I lift my head because applying pressure to my forehead causes my neck to shriek.

The doctor is correcting me.

All I really know is that I tested positive for the antibodies to the Lyme bacterium and the tests which indicated that are so inaccurate they're only ever relied upon by doctors who don't know just how unreliable they are.

Those tests mean nothing on their own. They only mean something when considered alongside symptoms. He tells me that Lyme disease is a clinical diagnosis and will remain so until some genius designs diagnostic tests that are less prone to whimsy.

Right. Got it. What?

I nod my head, or at least I would if I could move my neck, but I can't, so I just kind of bow forward slightly.

Nothing has changed for me. I mean, the reason the tests were done in the first place is because doctors were staring at a set of symptoms that at least one of them thought could be related to Lyme disease, so the criteria for a clinical diagnosis were met long ago, at least as far as I'm concerned.

But not as far as this doctor is concerned.

It seems Lyme disease has three stages and if I'd truly received a clinical diagnosis, I'd know what stage I'm in, but I don't know that.

This is the first I'm hearing of it.

Stage One (acute or early localized) normally occurs anywhere from a few days to a few weeks after a tick bite and can consist of flu-like symptoms such as aching joints, chills, fevers, fatigue, headaches, neck stiffness and sometimes a distinctive, expanding rash that may or may not look like a bull's eye. Secondary rashes may put in an appearance soon afterwards and can be located anywhere on the body. Conjunctivitis, swollen testes (for those of you who have them) and temporomandibular joint pain are also known Stage One symptoms.

Stage Two (early-disseminated) usually occurs anywhere from several weeks to several months after initial infection and its symptoms can include cardiac and neurological complications, arthritis, and wide-ranging visual problems.

Stage Three (late-disseminated) usually occurs months or years after initial infection and can include chronic arthritis especially of the large joints, rashes, and a whole host of neurological symptoms.

The three stages aren't cut and dried. There can be some overlap. A tossed salad effect.

The one thing that's for certain is the three weeks of antibiotics given to me when I was diagnosed with Lyme disease were the appropriate treatment for the acute stage only. They were a knee-jerk response to a positive test. Someone should've immediately followed up to determine which stage of the disease I was in and altered the treatment to suit the phase, but no one ever did.

This much is obvious to the doctor.

What's obvious to me is the top-down fracturing of my spine. I wriggle. I squirm. I can't find a comfortable position.

I want to cry, but I refuse to do that in front of a doctor.

Not even a nice one.

It seems there are a plethora of reasons to believe that I'm not in the acute stage of Lyme disease:

The first symptoms arrived more than five months prior to the disease being diagnosed and even then there were signs of neurological issues.

The radically slow heartbeat I suffered in the spring is characteristic of the second stage of the disease.

The sheer number and variety of neurological symptoms I developed over the past couple of months are typical of later stages of infection.

The hospitalization in June was likely due to an all-system breakdown caused by my organs being so full of infection they could no longer function properly.

The delayed onset of a Herx reaction usually occurs in the later stages of infection.

There may be other reasons, but I'm having trouble taking all of this in. My brain is swimming. It's trying to get away from my spine.

I'm with my brain on that one. I'd like to face my back to the wall and ram it until something catastrophic happens. I don't particularly care what. But I don't do this out of fear that I won't be able to handle the catastrophic thing when it arrives.

So I sit in my chair and silently scream, half-listening as the doctor lays out his case, which just happens to be my case. He's telling me that there's no possibility the disease was in the acute phase when it was diagnosed. At best it was in Stage Two, but the neurological symptoms are concerning and suggest that I may be in Stage Three of a disease that only has three stages.

Well, that's good, right? There's nowhere to go from here but up.

Or dead.

Take your pick.

I'm egging on death. It seems closer. Far easier to reach. And I have so little fight left in me that I need a goal that's within easy reach.

An interesting thing can happen when you expose Bb to antibiotics. Well, actually, several interesting things can happen, and I've already talked about toxins and Herx reactions and cystic forms, so now I'm going to talk about something a little different.

Bb has been shown to react to antibiotic exposure by converting into a cell-wall deficient form commonly known as an L-form. These L-forms look nothing like twizzles of yarn or microscopic boulders and they don't necessarily even look like Ls, despite their name.

L-forms are interesting for a couple of reasons. First, they're not the only type of cell to lack a wall. The cyst form of Bb doesn't have a cell wall either (and some would argue that the cysts are just variations on the L-form theme but, not surprisingly, there's no consensus on this), nor do native body cells — the ones that are supposed to be inside you — which is a really convenient thing for a bacterium to know if it wants to avoid a sound and sudden death.

Why?

Because the class of antibiotics traditionally used in the treatment of Lyme disease work, in whole or in part, by interfering with a bacterium's ability to form and/or maintain a structurally sound cell wall. When a bacterium can convert from having a cell wall to not having one, it's got an obvious advantage. These L-forms even retain their ability to generate both cell-wall deficient cysts and cell-wall intact spiral forms whenever they feel like it, making it yet another way in which Bb can survive just about everything that nature and pharmaceutical companies throw at it.

And while we're on the topic of interesting things these L-forms can do, I'd like to point out that they can join Bb's other forms in being able to enter native body cells and hide inside them until the coast is clear. Bb is particularly fond of hiding inside fibroblasts (which help form connective tissue), synovial cells (which form the fluid around your joints), and endothelial cells (which line your organs and blood vessels). And just to keep things interesting, they can even hide inside lymphocytes and macrophages — both immune system warriors — and move around your body hidden from your immune system inside its very own agents.

Your immune system can't get at them while they remain inside your body's own cells, at least not without destroying the native cells along with the invaders, something that looks and feels like an autoimmune attack. Nor can the antibiotics traditionally used against Lyme, so a class of antibiotics capable of entering cells and inhibiting the growth of Bb must be deployed.

And all because Bb is a bit of a trickster.

Safe to say a trickster isn't what my immune system signed on for.

The doctor is still talking and in theory I'm still listening.

In practice, I'm merely suffering.

He's telling me that cysts are filling my organs and possibly even my brain and my eyes.

At the very least, cyst-busting antibiotics will be needed in concert with conventional antibiotics to gain traction against the disease and the dual antibiotic treatment will likely last twelve to fifteen months, although I could get lucky and be clear of symptoms in as little as three months.

He doesn't think I'll get lucky.

There's also a chance treatment will fail. A big chance.

Oral antibiotics often fail in advanced Lyme. In which case, powerful intravenous (IV) antibiotics will be needed for a minimum of 90 days and possibly longer since treatment will have to continue until all symptoms resolve and there's no telling how long that might take.

The doctor is on his feet now.

He's on a mission.

He's telling me that it's important for me to leave his office armed with the information I need to make informed decisions about my health because I'm going to encounter a lot of ignorance among his colleagues. This catches me off guard and not because the doctor is openly criticizing the knowledge of his fellow doctors. I've done that myself too many times to be surprised to discover someone else shares my negative opinion. No, what catches me off guard is that after months of being ignored, insulted, and humiliated by doctors, I'm being told that I may have an antibiotic-resistant infection in my brain that will be extremely difficult, if not impossible, to eradicate. It's a sobering thought.

But it's not the only sobering thought. It seems that existing treatment guidelines for advanced Lyme disease don't allow for 90 days of IV treatment. If I want the treatment, I'll have to fight for it and most likely I'll fail to convince a specialist to sign off on that treatment in Canada, so I'll need to be prepared to leave the country — on my dime — and travel to the United States or Europe where that treatment is available. And it won't be cheap. Upwards of ten grand. It could even reach six figures before all is said and done.

And there's no guarantee of success.

The best the doctor before me can do is put me on a combination of two different oral antibiotics and hope that they'll be enough to eradicate the infection.

But he's skeptical and so am I. Why wouldn't I be? I'm so luckless these days it's almost funny.

This seems like a good point to talk about blebs, mostly because I don't want you leaving this chapter thinking that you know everything you need to know about Bb and its remarkable ability to survive anything and everything that's thrown at it.

Blebs (or granules) are an interesting spirochetal form, not least because nobody seems to be able to nail down exactly what function they fulfill.

What they do know is that when researchers view the spiral form of Bb under powerful microscopes, some of the spirals vibrate, then break into tiny fragments known as blebs. Most detectable Bb spirals have been shown to produce these tiny fragments along the surface of their bodies even when the bacteria aren't breaking apart.

So what are these blebs?

Originally researchers believed they were the end product of Bb's life cycle and some still persist in believing this, but there's evidence to suggest that they may be yet another one of Bb's survival forms and their formation is part of a strategy to help Bb, as a community, to weather the attacks of antibiotics and the immune system.

These blebs contain DNA — something that's essential when building a new generation — and it's possible that their primary purpose is to do just that. However, some researchers feel that instead of the next generation, these tiny fragments may be bits of outer surface proteins that are cleverly designed to be irresistible to the immune system's IgM antibodies. While these antibodies are preoccupied with hunting down the blebs, the spirochetes that generated them slip away unharmed.

Not a bad strategy.

And when you consider that these blebs are found everywhere in the body that Bb has colonized — including the central nervous system — you can see why some researchers believe they may be one of the many reasons why Lyme defies all attempts to defeat it and goes on to become a chronic and debilitating condition.

All of this brings us to the dirty secret that no one with Lyme ever wants to speak out loud: If Lyme disease isn't diagnosed and treated as soon as infection occurs — and before its survival forms have had a chance to develop — it may very well be incurable until new therapies are developed.

It hasn't escaped my notice that the Lyme doctor looks tired, worn out, defeated.

He's standing beside his chair, shifting between feet, and I suspect he's in pain although he never says so. Not directly, anyway.

As I fight to keep him in focus, he tells me that he's under investigation by a disciplinary committee at the College of Physicians and Surgeons of BC, specifically for diagnosing and treating Lyme disease patients with oral antibiotics beyond what existing guidelines allow for.

Apparently medical guidelines aren't actually guidelines, they're hard and fast rules. Break them and you're labeled a zealot. Or worse.

I make a note to add "guidelines" to the list of words that doctors define atypically.

The doctor tells me The College is asserting that he's behaving like an infectious disease specialist when he's licensed as a general practitioner, that he's diagnosing patients with Lyme when there's no evidence that many of these patients ever had that disease, and that he's treating the disease with oral antibiotics well beyond what's considered safe.

The doctor is defiant. He wouldn't be telling me all this if he wasn't. He won't back down, not willingly, anyway.

But he isn't a young man. He's far past the age where most people retire, and his health is failing due to the stress of fighting a licensing body he feels is wrong. It's clear that he won't be in practice much longer, no matter how strong his convictions are. Either death will take his body or The College will take his license. That much is obvious, even to me.

And once The College makes an example of this doctor, finding another willing to openly treat me for Lyme disease will be next to impossible.

This whole thing is a joke. A divine comedy.

I know only one thing for certain: I'm drowning and the only doctor willing to throw me a lifeline will soon have no choice but to let it go.

Unless I let go first.

I stumble out of his office. The floor tiles rise to slap the bottom of my feet at odd angles, sending me lurching between one wall and the next. As I make my way to the street, I'm certain of just two things:

1) The healthcare system has done more harm to me than an infected tick ever could.

2) If I continue to trust this ironically named system, I'll soon be dead.

BREAKING WITH CONVENTION

I make the arduous trip home from the doctor's office, over high mountain passes and through dark valleys, along a highway that rises and bends and curves far too often for my comfort.

I'm not the one driving, of course. My husband is the one doing that.

I can barely figure out what a car is these days, let alone how to operate one. I get confused by the lights and the dials and I can't even guess at what the rules of the road might be. Even if I could, I'd have to pull off the highway every dozen miles or so to rest my back on the cold, hard ground before getting back into the car and leapfrogging to the next resting point. It would take me days to complete a journey that should take hours. And I'd be a road hazard. A washed-out bridge. A patch of buckling pavement.

So I tilt the seat back and try to find a comfortable position. Sleep is too much to wish for. I wish for it anyway.

When we finally make it home, I go straight to bed and stay there for three days. Partly this is because the back of my neck feels like a balloon overfilled to the point of bursting and partly it's because my spine feels like it's splintering, but mostly it's because I can't cope with what the doctor has said.

It's locking up my brain. Every time I think about it, my mind tries to push the thought away.

But it won't go. It's urgent that I make a decision about my future before things get any worse.

Only I don't know what decision to make and it's paralyzing me.

I'm lying on the floor, trying to force air into lungs that are refusing to stretch. The air is scorching my airways. At least that's how it feels. More likely it's my airways that are scorching the air.

I'm tracing lines in the ceiling with tired eyes while trying hard to ignore the hum in my spine and the burbling at the base of my skull. I'm seeing more than just the wooden planks separating the rafters from the roof. I'm seeing thousands of tiny bubbles floating upwards, as if I'm looking at the world from inside a glass of ginger ale. At first these bubbles appear to be floating in the space between my eyes and the ceiling, but that's not the case. It turns out they're really rising over an opaque panel that breaks free and floats away. A second panel immediately replaces the first and that one too floats off, taking this new collection of bubbles with it.

Suddenly, I'm euphoric. I feel better than I've ever felt in my life. This surprises me, but it's such a glorious sensation that I willingly go with it until it takes an evil turn, intensifying beyond the point of overwhelming. It becomes critical that I shut the feeling down immediately, only I don't know how.

And I've run out of time.

My soul separates from my body. It floats several inches above where it should be and everything starts to move in slow motion.

Sight.

Sound.

Time.

I feel like I'm underwater. A fish lying prone at the bottom of a tank.

And yet I'm not underwater. I'm not under anything. I'm floating above my body like steam or smoke or a ribbon of mist.

There's a twinge at the base of my skull and every muscle in my body violently contracts. I'm aware of what's going on — I can sense it like a deer senses a wolf — but I'm no longer inside my body and I can't control anything it's doing.

I can't even connect what it's doing to me, not entirely.

I feel incredibly strange.

Like a mirage.

Or a whisper.

Or a ghost.

A ghost who's watching as the person I used to be dies.

I regain consciousness.

I'm inhumanly tired and I feel like I have the worst hangover of my life. At least the convulsing has stopped. I wonder when it stopped. I wonder why I don't know the answer.

Something is missing.

Time.

Memory.

It's hard to say what.

I sense movement to my left and gingerly turn my head. A naked man is strolling towards me, bathed in golden light. I don't recognize him. He has no features. His outline is approximate. So is his inline. His body is filled with swirling liquid light. I can see through him. I can see through everything.

The specter fades and so does my ocular omniscience.

I turn back to the ceiling and drift into nothing.

I come to again. Still tired, still boasting a nasty hangover. Nausea is flooding down the left side of my body.

It occurs to me that I forgot to mention why I'm lying on the floor. I'm lying here because pain is shooting out from between every single one of my vertebrae, making standing difficult and sitting impossible. Lying on a cold, hard floor doesn't resolve the problem, but it does make the pain bearable. Earlier I tried lying on my side, but my heart started to leap around like a frog in a shoebox, so I'm lying on my back hoping that my vertebrae rupture before things get much worse.

It's not that I don't have painkillers. I have the same kidney-blitzers I had before. But they don't even touch this kind of pain. I need morphine. Heroin. Laudanum. Any opiate will do. As long as the needle is clean and the dosages are pure. Well, not too pure. I don't want to be labeled a suicide.

I shouldn't be thinking like that. It's not helping the situation. It's hard to imagine what will. Which is why I'm thinking like that.

Until, suddenly, I'm not.

I come to again, no idea how long I was out. I open my eyes on a world that's tinged a lurid shade of red and I wonder what color the sun is. I consider looking, but even the light of a red sun will likely crack my skull, so instead I remain where I am and imagine the sun dripping great gobs of blood that splash when they hit the marigold earth.

I've got other things to worry about. Energy is shooting up my spine. What's surprising is the up.

Normally these bursts begin at the base of my skull and shoot downwards, so when one breaks with convention, it bears observing.

And what I'm observing is my body dissolving. It's more a sensation than a fact. I can see my chest rising and falling so I know it's still there. But where moments ago there was agony, now there's a cool breeze blowing through the place where my body once was. The absence extends from my neck to my toes, leaving an island of ice on my shin.

I can't move. There's nothing to move. At least nothing I can feel. I'd always assumed paralysis would feel like numbness, like when your foot falls asleep, or the dentist shoots Novocain into your gums. It doesn't feel like that. It doesn't feel like anything. Just absence. What the eye sees, the brain does not acknowledge.

So I return to tracing lines in the ceiling, hoping the absence will pass before it dawns on me how truly doomed I am.

It's hard to know what to do.

I can see no clear path forward.

It's difficult to imagine throwing in with a doctor who's clearly not going to be in practice for much longer and when he goes, then what? Who will take over my treatment? What doctor is going to draw a bull's eye on his or her forehead by taking over a roster of patients that the previous doctor was excused from the profession for trying to help?

I'm guessing that's a really short list.

But I have a prescription in my hand for three months of oral antibiotics. I can fill it any time I want and cross my fingers that I'll be cured by the time the meds run out. It's a gamble and luck hasn't exactly been on my side lately.

And then there's the problem that this treatment can cause serious liver problems and other complications. Who will bail me out if things start to go wrong? The doctor who shouted at me? The one who held my wrists and told me I was crazy? How about the doctor who suggested that I keep asking for help because I crave the attention? Or the specialist who is so busy he can't even schedule an appointment several months after receiving the referral?

No, I'm standing at the edge of a precipice with an inferno closing in on my heels. I can't go forward. I can't go backwards. All I can do is stay where I am.

But if I stay where I am I will surely burn.

All of this is academic. My options are really quite limited. I'm now so sick that I can't even imagine making it as far as the emergency room. And the trip would be pointless. There's no help to be found there, I've proven that much. No, I'm about as screwed as a person can get. I'm far sicker now than when I was admitted to the hospital months ago and steadily going downhill. I'm far sicker now, in fact, than I knew a human being could be and still survive.

But then maybe that's the point. Maybe I'm not going to survive. Maybe I've passed the point of no return and I'm about to learn firsthand what the afterlife is like.

I hope I come back as something cool. A solar eclipse or a blue morpho or an opal. Even a woolly mammoth. Nothing cuddly. That wouldn't be cool at all.

PART 2: PURGATORIO

At last we touched upon the lonely shore
that never yet has seen its waters sailed
by one who then returned to tell the tale.

— Dante Alighieri
Purgatorio

RAKING LEAVES

I'm slumped in a lawn chair on the front deck, my feet resting on the railing in front of me. The blur has cleared from my eyes and for the first time in days I can see blades of grass and stones and falling leaves. It's early autumn and most of the vegetables have been harvested from the garden my husband has somehow managed to keep weeded and watered this summer with little input from me.

He informs me that I've been fired as the Garden Commander.

I inform him that he doesn't have the authority to fire the Garden Commander.

He strides off, leaving me to contemplate the carrots, which still need pulling, and the frost-stricken tomatoes that really ought to be moved to the compost pile. I try, without success, to mentally guide the tomatoes over to the wheelbarrow.

Once again telekinesis is failing me.

Throughout this whole thing the only request I've made of God is that he bless me with a superpower. I think that's a reasonable request. More than reasonable. If God is going to send a disease to cripple me, the least he can do is give me a superpower to compensate for the wholesale destruction of my life. I promise not to abuse it. Honest.

My facial muscles are tight and the base of my skull is throbbing. A strange pressure is pushing down on the roof of my mouth, causing it to feel as though at any minute a tumor is going to break through and land on my tongue.

And I'm tired. So tired that I stop attempting to control the shaking in my thighs and instead rest my hands on my stomach.

Try as I might, I can't remember harvesting the beets. I stare at the spot in the garden where they should be, but all I see is churned-up soil and the pocks left by the heels of my boots. I must've harvested them already. When? I'm drawing a blank.

But then maybe *when* isn't nearly as important as *where*. I must've stashed the beets somewhere after I pried them from the ground, but where could that have been? The basement comes to mind, or the pump house, assuming I was operating on logic the day I did the work. If not, they could be in the linen closet or the bathtub or lined up along the eavestroughs. Any of these are possibilities, but none are sparking memories. That would be too easy. And nothing is easy these days.

I'll look for the beets later, if I remember, and likely I won't.

I need to stop this. I'm getting severely side-tracked and that's not helpful. The beets have nothing to do with why I'm sitting on my deck looking out over the garden. No, I'm sitting here because I'm watching my grandfather raking leaves off one of the grass paths that run between the garden beds. He's heaping them into a pile that he intends to burn later this afternoon and I don't waste my energy asking him whether he's bothered to get a permit. He wouldn't answer me if I did.

So instead I watch the rake scratching the damp grass and study my grandfather, who is wearing the same dusk-blue utility coat he's worn for doing yard work for as long as I can remember. He's tall and strong and possesses a regal bearing that seems to fly in the face of his advancing years. True, his movements are stiff, and there's a slight shake in his left hand, but it's not nearly as pronounced as the tremors rattling my thighs and, by extension, the railing surrounding the deck. My grandfather is holding strong against the vagaries of age and I'm cracking under the weight of this relentless disease.

But I wouldn't wish what's happening to me on him. I wouldn't wish it on anyone.

Still, I can't help but wonder why my grandfather is wasting his time raking all those leaves into a burn-pile when he could just as easily be spreading them out over the unharvested carrots, saving me a lot of effort. That's a selfish thought, I know, but it's hard to sit here in my thirties watching a man in his seventies doing a chore that I should be doing myself.

I consider shouting something to my grandfather about the carrots, just to see if I can get him to alter his plans at my request, but my jaw is aching and my tongue has already made several urgent requests that I not move it any more than absolutely necessary, so I don't press my luck. Instead I wonder whether I can control the shaking and the pain and the dysfunction long enough to help him out.

Christ, what am I thinking?

I'm not thinking; that's the problem.

Any attempt to help my grandfather would be pointless.

There's no way I can help a man who's been dead for nearly 20 years.

WARM OCEAN BREEZES

Say what you will about Bb, it's a very sociable bacterium and when it travels it likes to bring along its friends. It's estimated that anywhere between 15 and 60 percent of Lyme patients in endemic regions of the northeastern United States contract a second tick-borne pathogen when they contract Bb, depending entirely on which researchers are doing the estimating. There are even recorded cases of patients hitting the jackpot, receiving three or more infections from a single tick bite.

Now that's bad luck.

It's not yet known what percentage of Canadian Lyme disease sufferers have co-infections with other tick-borne illnesses and it likely won't be known for a very long time due largely to a lack of research into the subject. For now, it's enough to know that many Canadian Lyme disease patients are being treated for co-infections, although not necessarily in this country.

Tick-borne infections are so little understood here that testing for suspected tick-borne infections often begins and ends with Lyme disease.

If it even begins.

Co-infections are rarely considered.

Of these co-infecting organisms, babesia (a parasite that attacks red blood cells), anaplasma (a bacterium that attacks white blood cells), and bartonella-like organisms (a class of bacteria normally associated with infections in cats) are the most common. But mycoplasma, tick-borne encephalitis, ehrlichia, *Chlamydia trachomatis*, Rocky Mountain spotted fever, tularemia, and dozens of viruses can all be contracted from the same ticks that carry Lyme disease.

It's even possible to contract organisms not yet known to medical science.

Say what you will about these tiny arachnids, ticks do themselves proud as infection-breeding machines by incubating more pathogenic organisms than any other known vector and someday researchers will succeed in fully mapping the impressive variety of pathogens that live in their guts.

But someday isn't today.

I'm looking in the mirror and I don't like what I'm seeing.

Nor do I understand it. The left side of my face is frozen and drooping as if it started to melt, then solidified. When I press my fingers against my cheek, my face doesn't register the touch, but my fingers register a material that doesn't feel much like human flesh. It feels more like rubber or possibly like raw chicken. Very strange.

It doesn't usually get this bad. Normally, that cheek feels tight and there's a tingling numbness like when a sleeping foot begins to wake up. If I tap my index finger against my cheekbone, there's a muffled sensation, as if padding has been placed between my finger and the skin. Yet most of the time, the muscles continue to function despite the altered sensation. Sometimes they flutter or twitch. Sometimes a sting streaks across the numbness like a comet racing across the midnight sky. At other times there's a delay between when I start to smile and when that smile abruptly kicks in — just on one side of my face — making me look momentarily insane. But, for the most part, I can grimace or frown or even blow kisses if I want to. I just don't want to.

Then there are days like today. Days when the pressure at the base of my skull is so intense it feels as if my head is going to pop off my neck like a dandelion flower forced from its stem by a determined thumb. On those days the numbness starts at the base of my skull and wraps around behind my ear where it's anchored to the bone by razor-sharp spurs. My cheek goes numb and droops and there's a feeling of incredible tension, as if my cheek is being reeled in by my nose. I look like a hound dog. Half of my face does, anyway.

And I press my fingers to my cheek. Mesmerized. Horrified. I'm thinking just one thing: This is what my face will feel like when I die.

Of those Lyme patients who have co-infections with other tick-borne pathogens, it's estimated that up to two-thirds are infected with a species of babesia. Babesia is a parasite that infects and destroys red blood cells. It's North America's answer to malaria, but unlike malaria, which is transmitted by mosquitoes, babesia is transmitted by ticks.

The same ticks that carry Lyme disease.

On its own, babesia can cause balance problems, headaches, fatigue, anorexia, muscle and joint pain, chest compression, breathing problems, high fevers, shaking chills, nausea, malaise, drenching night sweats, persistent coughs, and/or vomiting. When Lyme disease and babesia share the same host, the two organisms act symbiotically, creating a rather messy clinical picture that's more severe, longer in duration, and has a greater number of symptoms than when either illness arrives alone. Although highly variable, those symptoms can include air hunger, severe headaches, anemia, CNS disturbances, and inflammation of the spinal cord in addition to the symptoms listed above.

And get this: Many experts believe that in order to successfully treat Lyme disease, you must first cure the babesia infection or Bb will fail to resolve no matter how many antibiotics you throw at it.

And that's a problem.

In order to dispatch babesia, you must first determine that it's present and that can be a difficult thing to do since many instances of babesiosis produce few or mild symptoms that are often mistakenly attributed to Lyme disease. Complicating matters is the testing for babesia, which isn't as comprehensive or as reliable as one would hope.

I haven't eaten for days. I can't stand the way food smells. Everything is fragrant to the point of overwhelming. To the point of pain.

The odor that dairy products emit is repellant, so is the stench from wheat, soy, chicken, and grapes. It's not that they smell rancid. They smell like what they are, only amplified to an unappetizing extreme. I mean, there's a reason they don't make incense in these fragrances.

If I try to eat anything with an aroma, the nausea is overwhelming. Sometimes I throw up. Sometimes not. The only way I can avoid all this is to eat scentless food. Rye crackers. Raw vegetables. Boiled rice. I have the diet of an ascetic.

And Lyme hasn't just been monkeying with my sense of smell. It's also been altering my sense of taste. I guess that makes sense. If your sense of smell goes wonky then it's likely that your sense of taste will follow suit. Any seven-year-old can tell you that. But you'd think taste and smell would be affected in the same way. At least I would. Yet things don't taste like overwhelming versions of their former selves. They taste strange. Cheese tastes like metal. Eggs taste like mushrooms. Mushrooms taste like vomit. Cherries taste like beer.

Strawberries taste like strawberries. Go figure.

Babesia is relatively new to medical science. The first human case of babesiosis wasn't identified in North America until 1969 and of the dozen or so babesia species that have so far been identified, only three are known to routinely infect humans. Of those, two are of concern to Canadians: *Babesia microti* (central and eastern Canada) and WA-1 (western Canada).

Tests haven't yet been developed for all of the known species of babesia and researchers have expressed concerns that species other than the dominant three may also be causing human infections, something future research will one day shed light on. For now, only the most common strains are tested for, so if you contract babesia, hope that it's of the microti or WA-1 variety; otherwise, you're out of luck in the testing department.

To make things really interesting, the symptoms of babesia have been known to arrive long after initial infection, something that can also be said of Lyme disease. Both illnesses are known, in some cases, to show few (or no) symptoms when they first arrive and can remain mostly or entirely asymptomatic for extended periods of time — weeks, months, even years — before popping up in full-blown glory. When Lyme disease isn't present, babesia often resolves on its own without the patient ever being aware that they were infected.

When Lyme is present, however, it's a different story entirely.

It says something about the state of medical knowledge in Canada that the only doctor who would ever broach the topic of Lyme's co-infections is the one I tracked down through improper channels who immediately had me tested for the most common ones, including babesia. Not one other doctor even seemed to be aware that ticks could transmit several infecting (and non-infecting) agents with a single bite. Asking any other doctor questions about babesia, for instance, inspired the sort of reaction I'd expect to get if I were to suddenly bounce a nickel off a stranger's forehead.

Not exactly confidence inspiring.

And babesia is by far the most common co-infection.

Imagine the reaction I would've gotten if I'd asked about any other co-infecting organism.

A vegetarian for more than twenty years, my cravings for meat are now so powerful I'd be willing to kill a pig with my bare hands if that'd get it onto my dinner plate any faster.

The urgency of this craving is deceptive.

It implies hunger, but I often can't eat more than a bite before my stomach insists it's full. I perpetually feel like I've gorged on a twelve-course meal when I haven't taken so much as a single bite. So I force myself to eat whether my body wants the food or not. That seems like the responsible thing to do, but it takes a lot of willpower.

And I don't have a lot of willpower.

I stand in front of the open refrigerator and stare blankly at its contents. There's nothing inside that interests me and I can't think of what to eat in the absence of interest. I try stuffing the fridge full of my favorite foods, only to discover that they no longer hold any appeal.

Maybe I'll eat the air.

It smells and tastes like what it is.

Most of the time, anyway. Although, come to think of it, sometimes the air is shot through with sudden, strong odors that no one else seems able to detect. Usually the smells are of burning rubber or rotting food or sewage.

Never of jasmine or lilac.

So then maybe I shouldn't try eating the air. But since that'll get me no further ahead than I am now, maybe I should go on a hunger strike instead.

At least then my body and my mind will be in sync.

No discussion of Bb would be complete without mentioning biofilms. Although they get very little press when it comes to Lyme disease, they are very important.

Bb can exist in something called a biofilm community, which essentially means that instead of each tiny bacterium running around inside its host like a rogue commando, it can hook up with a bunch of its friends and together they can surround themselves with a protective gel-like blob. Inside this blob, known as a biofilm, they live peacefully, protected from any number of environmental stressors — including antibodies and antibiotics — which must first penetrate the gel before they can attack the organisms hidden within it.

Easier said than done. Antibiotics often can't penetrate far enough into the biofilm to get at the sequestered bacteria. Nor can antibodies.

Yet these biofilm communities do more than protect their member organisms from attack. They also allow them to swap information back and forth like gossip at a neighborhood barbeque. And by information, I mean genetic information, which individual Bb cells can exchange between each other and any co-infecting organisms that may also be ensconced in the biofilm with them, such as babesia.

You read that right. There's evidence to suggest that Bb may be able to swap genetic information back and forth with an unrelated organism — a protozoan, not a bacterium — altering both pathogens in a way that makes them stronger and harder to defeat.

And then there's the biofilm itself. This gel-like sanctuary comprises extracellular DNA (eDNA), which is exactly what it sounds like: DNA that's not a part of any bacterium, protozoan, or virus the biofilm may contain, but which exists outside of these organisms in the biofilm itself where it does several things, including increasing resistance to environmental stressors and stabilizing the biofilm's structure.

Now this eDNA is an intrinsic part of the biofilm, so if you were thinking that the gel-like blob protecting these sequestered organisms was an inert substance, think again. It's far from that. It's more of a willing accomplice. And it has the manners of the town drunk. Biofilms can burp and they can burp a lot. And what they're burping are the toxic byproducts of the creatures (bacteria, protozoa, viruses) living inside them. It's theorized that these byproducts are a major cause of Lyme's more persistent symptoms. Of course, lots of things are theorized as being major causes of Lyme's persistent symptoms. That's another one of the many joys of trying to get a handle on an emerging disease. Hypotheses abound. Cold, hard facts are in short supply.

Anyway, these biofilm communities inspire awe. In order to kill an entrenched Bb infection, antibiotics must first penetrate the biofilm, but in all likelihood they'll fail to get far enough to pose any real threat to the organisms sequestered within it. Those that do get far enough can find themselves faced with a form of Bb that's evolved from what it was before it entered the community thanks to Bb's innate proclivity for antigenic variation as well as its wanton swapping of genetic information with unrelated organisms.

When you also take into consideration that Bb can be present inside the biofilm in not just its spiral form, but also in its cell-wall deficient cyst and L-forms — both of which are challenging to defeat under normal circumstances — the only possible reason the ancient Greeks didn't write a myth about this stuff is because they hadn't invented high-powered microscopes. Had they, we'd be learning about Bb in high school alongside tales of Pandora and Prometheus and that dude who went searching for The Golden Fleece.

I'm considering getting nostalgic over how smell and taste and lack of appetite once affected my ability to eat because they're the least of my worries these days.

Swallowing used to be as simple as having the urge but, like a metal gear long exposed to warm ocean breezes, the mechanism that allows me to swallow moves grudgingly, if at all. You swallow more times in a day — more times in an hour — than you can possibly be aware of until the day your ability to swallow becomes seriously compromised. That's when you find yourself making hard decisions, like choosing to clear the saliva from your mouth by drooling it onto a towel like a dying puppy in the hopes that when it comes time to eat maybe, just maybe, that gear will be rested enough for you to choke down some nutrients before you starve to death.

And starving to death is becoming a real possibility. My weight is falling faster than a stone down a well. This is the first time in my life that losing weight doesn't register as a triumph.

I'm so hungry I'm clawing at food. But the only way I can get any nutrients is to dump liquids into my esophagus without letting them come in contact with the roof of my mouth or the back of my tongue, both of which balk at the mere suggestion of anything moving over their surfaces.

Air is bad enough. Food causes them to freak. Which causes me to freak.

So my husband uses a blender to liquefy whatever I'm contemplating eating so that I can lie on the couch and pour it into my mouth with my tongue firmly clamped between my teeth to prevent it from recoiling down my throat.

This is trickier than it sounds. I can't actually feel my teeth or the tip of my tongue, so the only way I know that my teeth are firmly clamping my tongue and not biting straight through it is to do a double-check with my fingers.

And then I dump. I either swallow or choke. Often I do both.

I can't do the whole dumping thing sitting up and tipping my head back because I can't actually sit up for longer than a few minutes at a time and even if I could, my neck won't bend back. It certainly won't bend forward. It can manage sideways in a pinch but that's not terribly helpful when you're trying to dump liquidized food into your esophagus.

The whole dumping process isn't flawless, and there are times when my jaw is locked so tight not even a diamond-tipped crowbar could pry it open, complicating things further. But, when you get right down to it, the process doesn't have to be flawless, it just has to be possible. And that's where it succeeds brilliantly.

I don't fill the prescription for the oral antibiotics. When it gets right down to it, I'm afraid to start down that road, knowing that the doctor who wrote the prescription won't be around to provide me with more or different antibiotics as the situation demands. And I don't trust local doctors to bail me out if things go wrong, not after they've failed me so many times in the past. Nor do I have the strength to travel eight hours by car to meet with a hypothetical specialist in some distant city so that I can suffer the indignity of fighting for the right to receive IV antibiotics for a duration that exceeds what's recommended in the existing treatment guidelines for Lyme disease. You don't have to be a genius to figure out how that conversation will end.

Then there's that very voguish question of antibiotic resistance. The antibiotic I was treated with earlier this year isn't a possibility for treatment now. It might have done the job if it'd been prescribed for several months or years instead of several weeks, but if you've learned nothing else about Bb, you must surely have learned that it's a highly adaptable organism, one that will have switched up its surface proteins and mutated into survival forms in an effort to be less susceptible to the antibiotic that was already sent in after it.

That antibiotic can't be used against Bb again. At least not in me.

So I have a prescription for two other antibiotics, one conventional and the other a cyst-buster. If I take them and then find myself abruptly, brutally, cut off after three months — something that's very likely — then that's two more antibiotics down the tubes with no guarantee of a cure to show for it. If more treatment is required, it'll have to be without the three antibiotics already used and then the possibility starts to become very real that I may run out of antibiotics before the infection is defeated.

Then what? How do I win the battle against a superbug that I was complicit in creating?

And I certainly don't have the money to pursue treatment in Europe or the United States, even if I were inclined in that direction. And I'm not. It seems wrong to be driven out of my own country to pursue medical treatment when I've been told my entire life that universal healthcare is the birthright of all Canadians. Except, apparently, me.

And then there's that little voice in the back of my mind. That obnoxious, nagging little voice I know so well. It's telling me that taking the advice of a doctor who is under review for his atypical treatment of patients just like me may not be the wisest move I'll ever make. I mean, the folks doing the persecuting aren't idiots, right? They wouldn't be doing what they're doing without having a solid foundation for their concerns, would they?

These questions aren't rhetorical, although perhaps they should be.

My fingernails have recorded the recent upheavals in much the same way that the Earth's crust pleats in response to the awesome forces of nature. What I'm trying to say is that my fingernails are now horribly deformed. They look like the surface of rocks that have been shaped then reshaped by the violent stop-start motion of ancient glaciers. These undulations vary in width and frequency, yet together they look like a barcode cut into bone. The effect is more pronounced on my toenails, but those I can hide in socks. My fingernails I actually have to see and every glimpse takes my breath away.

I don't know what process causes fingernails to grow and I don't want to know. I can't imagine I'll find much comfort in the answer. Whatever that process is, it's faltering, badly. The proof is in plain sight at the end of my fingers. It's really quite a sight. Gnarly fingernails look remarkably like something you'd expect to see on a demon. Or a dragon. Or a troll.

There are days when I feel like a refugee from a fairy tale that I neglected to read as a child. I wish I had read it. I'd really like to know how this story ends.

BLOATING LIKE A DEAD WHALE

It's hard to navigate though life without any bearings.

I don't know where hallways lead because, basically, I've lost the ability to extrapolate beyond what I can see. If I enter a building and lose sight of the entrance, I have no idea how to get back out. I suppose I could retrace my steps, but that would require me to remember what they were and I can't, so I either ask for directions or fake that I know where I'm going. I usually opt for faking.

Grocery stores are the worst. Just trying to pick up a few groceries is like treasure hunting in a labyrinth. Every aisle I peer down, every display case I encounter, is filled with a chaotic jumble of contrasting shapes and colors, none of it meaningful. Overhead signs announce what products can be found down each aisle, but there's an assumption being made that I'll be able to match an object to its name — and worse — that I'll be able to see "Flour" listed on a sign and know that baking soda is down that same aisle. But I don't know that. The only way I have to find the baking soda is to trip down every aisle until I either find it or forget what I'm looking for. Sometimes I succeed, mostly I don't.

I consider myself successful if I manage to locate half of the things on my list. Come to think of it, I didn't fare much better when I had a fully functioning brain.

I'm at the grocery store now.

It takes me an hour to buy a loaf of bread.

It doesn't help that I'm fully aware that a seven-year-old armed with a handful of change could march into this same store and come out with the bread in five minutes. At the age of 38 there's no guarantee I can do the same. The worst of it is that although I've lost the ability to function as a competent adult, I haven't lost the knowledge that I used to. Nor have I lost the understanding that the task I'm struggling to complete is a simple one.

But it isn't simple. It's so complex it's verging on impossible. Once in the store, I forget why I'm here until prompted. I fail to recognize the loaf of bread as being a loaf of bread until my husband points out the obvious and then grabs my arm as I head for the door, guiding me back to the check-out so that I can pay for it. And I stand there stupidly. I don't remember how the transaction goes. I don't understand that I'm required to give the cashier money.

When I finally clue in, I can't figure out if the money in my hand is enough to pay for the bread. The cashier points to a five-dollar bill and suggests that I hand it over, but then she goes and complicates things by asking me a question and I stop fumbling so that I can ask her to repeat it. I do this several times, but I still can't grasp what she's asking, so I shrug my shoulders in defeat. My husband takes the money from my hand and the cashier hands him the change. I wait expectantly for what comes next, not quite grasping that the transaction has concluded.

Sometimes this embarrasses me.

The rest of the time I'm so determined to make a success of what I'm doing that I plug away at it no matter how many times I need to be prompted or how many mistakes I make.

Maybe I should consider this training for when I'm 85.

Of course, at the rate I'm going, it's doubtful I'll be making it to 45.

I don't recall being bitten by a tick, but since that's how Lyme and its co-infections enter the human body, evidence strongly suggests that at some point prior to January 2007 my blood provided a tasty meal to at least one tick.

In eastern Canada, public health officials have fingered the black-legged tick, *Ixodes scapularis*, (commonly known as the deer tick) as the primary vector for Bb in that region while in western Canada, the western black-legged tick, *Ixodes pacificus*, gets the nod.

You don't need me to tell you this. This information is widely available in any number of publications put out by public health agencies across our fair country. And since I've lived in both Ontario and British Columbia, conventional wisdom says that one of these two ticks did the honors.

Or not.

Lyme information widely available in Canada almost exclusively names these two ticks as the prime suspects in Bb infections, but several studies suggest that other ticks may be, at least in part, to blame for the spread of the bacterium across the country. It seems Bb has been found thriving in dozens of tick species other than the two Ixodes mentioned above, including *Amblyomma, Argas, Dermacentor, Haemaphysalis, Ornithodorus* and other species of *Ixodes* ticks, examples of which have all been found in Canada, either because they've established permanent populations here or because they've been carried here by migratory birds. There's also evidence to suggest that mosquitoes, biting flies, fleas and even mites may be able to host and possibly even transmit Bb infections, but so far the data on these possible vectors have been inconclusive.

Such is the joy of dealing with a subject for which research is still in its infancy.

Studies have mostly focused on the role of Ixodes ticks in the transmission of Bb infections in this country. Until comprehensive research has been conducted into other possible vectors, the claim that *I. scapularis* and *I. pacificus* are responsible for most infections in Canada is more of an assumption than a verifiable fact.

Only time, and research, will tell how accurate that assumption truly is.

I'm standing on the sidewalk in front of the bank, trying to determine how I came to be standing on the sidewalk in front of the bank. Someone walks up to me and strikes up a conversation, which has nothing to do with the bank I'm standing in front of and this confounds me.

I can't see the speaker's face, so I'm having trouble making out who she is. It's not that she has no features. It's just that those features are hidden behind fluttering gauze. Not literally, of course, but the gauze might as well be there. I can't make out her eyes, her nose, or her chin — or how they fit together to form a visage — but I can see non-facial features just fine.

Hair.

Clothes.

Shoes.

It's just unfortunate that I have a lifelong history of identifying people by their faces. So I'm listening and watching in the desperate hope that some phrase or gesture or article of clothing will clue me in to whether the person before me is a neighbor, a friend, a total stranger, or my mother.

I'm not asking for a miracle. I don't need to know the exact identity of the speaker. I just need to get it in the ballpark so that when it's my turn to speak I'll have some idea whether my response should be intimate or vague or something in between. How well does this person know me?

The problem with venturing into public is that I spend so much time trying to figure out where I am and who I'm talking to that it's hard to get anything meaningful done. Instead of, say, buying a carton of milk or picking up a package at the post office, my energy is spent faking my way through conversations with nameless, faceless apparitions.

I want to go home, even though things aren't perfect there either. There are days when I can't figure out how to unlock a door or punch a telephone number into a keypad. I can't grasp how a calculator works, how to get a letter into an envelope, or even how to tie my shoelaces.

And then there are childproof containers. Eventually I figure out how to open one, but not because I solve the mechanical riddle at its heart. No, I open it because I own a hammer and after repeated attempts to coax the lid off the bottle fail, the hammer succeeds.

I feel safe at home, though, mostly because few people venture down the rural road where I live, greatly increasing the odds that I'll be able to identify whomever has made the mistake of trying to enter into a conversation with me. I've learned to identify my neighbors by their vehicles, their clothing, or their hairstyles. I no longer need to see their faces to know who they are unless I meet them in town. Then all bets are off. Context is everything.

Today I've ventured into town to undertake some chore that's currently escaping my mind — a chore which may or may not have something to do with the bank I'm standing in front of — and now I've been cornered by an apparition who won't go away.

Who is this person I'm talking to?

And why should I care?

Without faces, people are as real to me as B-movie specters and so I don't always take the time to figure out who they are. Sometimes I wander off mid-sentence. Sometimes I start talking about supernovas or string theory or the contents of my vacuum. Sometimes I say nothing and wait for the apparition to give up.

That's the thing about apparitions: You can mess with them all you want without worrying about their feelings. Apparitions don't have feelings. How can they? They're dead or they wouldn't be apparitions. I'm not sure how high on the logic meter that thought ranks, but really, who cares?

This mangled attempt at a conversation is hitting the point where I normally lapse into silence. Only today I think it might be important to figure out who the apparition is, so I give it a try.

But I'm flailing. Badly. And so I start babbling about the ancient disaster of a catalpa tree that's slowly rotting by the entrance to the post office and pretend to care whether it lives or dies. In this way I buy myself some time.

It's too bad I don't buy enough of it.

Ticks like to hang out in grassy fields, brush, wooded areas, forest clearings and anywhere else where there's lots of low-lying vegetation and copious amounts of leaf litter.

And so do I.

In fact, that's a pretty bang-on description of where I live. If you look out any window of my home, you'll see grassy fields, brush, wooded areas and/or forest clearings — not to mention copious amounts of leaf litter — so it's really no wonder that two creatures with similar habitat preferences would one day meet.

Since I don't remember being bitten by a tick on my property or anywhere else, we're going to have to take it on faith that home turf is where the encounter occurred. I could've just as easily come in contact with my assailant(s) on one of my hiking trips through the wonderfully scenic parks and trails in the Vancouver area.

Now, maybe it sounds a little strange to pick up an infection from a tick in an urban area, but the majority of Lyme-infected ticks in this province have traditionally been found within heavily populated areas in the southwestern region of the province, including Vancouver and the Lower Mainland, the Fraser Valley, the Sunshine Coast, and Vancouver Island, where temperate winters and high humidity make for excellent tick habitat. The less populated Kootenay region, where I live, is also known to have its fair share of Lyme-infected ticks.

The fact is, many people infected with Bb pick up the bacterium in their own backyards, in neighborhood parks, or along footpaths in the urban and suburban areas in which they live, work, and play. So who knows where I was bitten? Vancouver's Stanley Park is as much a possibility as the forest clearing in the Rocky Mountains that is my backyard.

Certainly, the chances of contracting Lyme are much higher if you live in an endemic area and indeed I do, so in trying to pinpoint ground zero for my infection, I'm going to have to go with my own property in the Kootenays unless some compelling evidence turns up to supersede that theory.

Let's step back in time for a moment.

Until 1997, Long Point in southern Ontario was the only place in Canada officially recognized as having an endemic population of Lyme-infected ticks. And by "endemic" I mean that all three stages of a tick's life cycle are found in an area over two or more consecutive years.

How things have changed.

Ticks known to harbor Bb have now established permanent populations in many areas of southern Ontario and Quebec, Nova Scotia, southeastern Manitoba and British Columbia. In fact, BC is so hospitable to these tiny arachnids, it's estimated that three-quarters of the tick species found in Canada make their home in this province and most of those are capable of transmitting pathogens that can cause illness in humans and animals.

Still, the endemic areas listed above are only the ones recognized by public health officials.

It turns out that ticks couldn't care less where officials say they should be.

As Lyme disease sufferers across this country will attest, you can contract Lyme in any number of locales that haven't yet been given a golden checkmark by these officials. (But then many of those sufferers have themselves not been given the golden checkmark by public health officials. We'll get to that in a minute.)

A 2009 report noted that a whopping 85 percent of Ontarians who acquired Lyme disease inside that province between 2002 and 2006 had not visited any of the endemic areas defined by public health officials. Now I don't mean to nitpick, but when only 15 percent of a province's Lyme sufferers acquire their infections in known endemic areas, it's probably a safe bet that there's a problem with the way endemic areas are being defined.

Just saying.

Did I mention that the apparition who has me cornered in front of the bank is speaking in hieroglyphics? No, really. You know what hieroglyphics look like, right? Well, imagine the ancient Egyptians actually saying those symbols out loud and that'll give you a good idea what I'm hearing right now.

Under different circumstances, this could make a great drinking game.

Under these circumstances, I'm stymied.

I haven't yet figured out who the apparition is and I can only guess at what she might be talking about. I hope that my brain gets with the translating soon; otherwise, I'll be forced to wander off like a lost cow.

So I concentrate.

I try to find a hook.

A root word.

Who am I kidding?

The nameless, faceless apparition is speaking in smudges and gaps and I can wring no meaning from those. I mean, I once tried to learn Morse code from the instructions on the outside of a cereal box, but I never really got past S-O-S and what I'm hearing now isn't that.

I don't know what it is.

Whale song.

Verbal sign language.

Tribal drumbeats.

All useless to anyone not schooled in their meanings.

I ask the apparition to repeat what she just said, not because I think hearing a jumble of nonsensical sounds a second time will unlock their meaning, but because I'm trying to buy myself time to figure out how to escape this conversation without letting on just how defective I am.

So I pretend to be distracted by the sound of an approaching car. Only I'm not really pretending. The auditory plane has been flattened like a raccoon on a highway rendering everything I'm hearing into a noise pancake. I don't seem to be able to distinguish between directed sound and ambient noise and so I'm having trouble determining which sounds are coming from the apparition and which are coming from a passing car.

It's not immediately obvious and it really should be. I'm so frustrated I want to punch the bank. Better yet, I'd like the problem to do me a ginormous favor and just move on. But it doesn't ever just move on.

And it isn't limited to what I'm hearing. My speech is often so tangled, it sounds like spaghetti. I'm never sure what's going to come out of my mouth until I hear it, leaving me just as perplexed as whomever I'm speaking to.

Sometimes words come out properly formed. Sometimes they stick like gum in hair. I stammer or stutter or slur. I garble words and speak gibberish. I leave complicated words half-spoken or I bog down on tense. Strange gaps crop up mid-sentence and leapfrog through paragraphs, landing in unpredictable places that cause sentences to buckle or lurch.

At other times I speak so slowly you could recite the balcony scene from *Romeo and Juliet* in the space of time it takes me to say my own name. And I lose words, causing sentences to hang helplessly in the air like flags on a gust-free day. Even when I do manage to spit a sentence out, my brain connects thoughts in unpredictable ways, cramming five incomplete ideas together in a single malformed sentence that no one, not even me, can understand.

This is what happens now. And I'm baffled. I know what I've said is wrong, but I can't put my finger on what specifically is wrong about it, leaving me powerless to make a correction. The apparition knows what I've said is wrong too and is slowly backing away. I'm not sure what to do. I don't dare speak for fear of what might come out.

There are times when all of this strikes me as hilarious. This isn't one of those times.

Let's take a look at why ticks and humans are colliding with increasing frequency.

As urban populations swell, houses and people spill out onto land that until recently remained under nature's sole dominion. Subdivisions sprawl across farmland, shopping malls perch on former wetlands, and grassy plains lie crushed beneath concrete and steel and pavement. Add to this the growing number of Canadians fleeing urban and suburban life for calmer existences on small acreages or in cottages nestled in the woods and, well, you get the picture.

Did we really believe that our incursions into nature would carry no consequences?

Yes, we really did. And we still do. It's one of the many quirks of human nature.

This unrelenting expansion into nature is bringing us increasingly closer to its denizens and included amongst those are the deer that have been roaming this continent longer than we have. Couple this with a dramatic reduction in the number of wolves, mountain lions, and other predators that traditionally kept deer populations under control and you get an excellent opportunity for humans to become infected with the sorts of diseases that normally infect deer.

Lyme is just one of those diseases.

Also in the mix is the rise of coyote populations in areas where foxes have traditionally reigned, something that's notable because when the coyotes move in, the foxes move out and those retreating foxes have traditionally done an excellent job of keeping rodent populations under control. Their absence — and indeed a general decline in biodiversity — causes a surge in the number of rodents zipping around which in turn causes a surge in the chances of humans contracting Lyme.

Several other factors have caused the distribution of ticks to bloat like a dead whale in recent years and, in British Columbia, the fragmentation of formerly vibrant old-growth forests is certainly playing a role. The lumber industry has not only reshaped the landscape of this province, it's also reshaped the health of its citizens. As the ancient, hulking trees that once defined BC are struck down in an effort to profit from the world's seemingly insatiable demand for wood and paper products, vast swaths of brush have replaced the once vibrant ecologies those forests contained. And all that brush is the perfect habitat for rodents, deer, and the ticks that feed on both.

This alone is enough to ensure a dramatic increase in tick populations, but it isn't alone. Conservation and rehabilitation efforts are also in the loop. Although positive on the whole, such efforts require human intervention into natural systems, something that will never be without consequences, since they mean tinkering with nature in a way that humans deem positive. Nature may or may not agree, so instead of correcting a human-made imbalance, conservation and rehabilitation efforts can potentially unbalance an ecosystem in a whole new way that may not come to our attention for years or decades down the road.

And then there's climate change.

Yes, the topic none of us can avoid, no matter how desperately we'd like to, is having a dramatic impact on the distribution of ticks as southern regions of Canada warm to the point where permanent populations of ticks can thrive.

And thrive they do.

Just a few decades ago, random ticks would turn up in regions of BC and other provinces where they'd never before been seen, but more often than not they would succumb to the brutal winter temperatures before they could establish permanent populations. That's no longer the case in an increasing number of areas where these random ticks are not only surviving the cold, they're breeding. And in breeding, they're gaining lasting footholds in territories that just a few years ago would have been unthinkable.

One recent study found tick species known to harbor Bb alive and well as far north as the Yukon. Another reported that *Ixodes scapularis* ticks are expanding their territory so rapidly that within just over a decade, three-quarters of Canadians will be living in areas with established tick populations capable of carrying Lyme bacteria. Even ultra conservative government-funded researchers have had no choice but to acknowledge that the range of infected ticks in Canada is rapidly expanding and will continue to do so for the foreseeable future.

That raises the question of how these ticks are arriving in these new regions.

I mean, ticks don't get around much. Without assistance, your average tick would be born, live and die in an area smaller than the average baseball diamond. But ticks do get assistance.

They hitch rides on the vertebrates they attach themselves to in their quest to obtain the blood they need to propel their life cycles. When these ticks attach themselves to rodents, they don't travel very far since rodents generally don't travel more than about 30 square meters in their lifetimes. But when they attach themselves to deer, dogs, or humans they really go places.

Deer have a range of approximately four kilometers.

Dogs and humans range even farther.

However, it's our feathered friends who range the farthest. When ticks attach themselves to migrating birds, the sky, as they say, is the limit. Well, actually, 425 kilometers is the generally accepted limit for how far a migrating bird is likely to carry an infected tick beyond a known endemic area.

But the generally accepted limit may not be telling the whole story.

If the ticks capable of carrying Bb have been found in northern Alberta and the Yukon — and they have — it's safe to say they can be found anywhere in this country. Birds have historically been known to carry ticks from one continent to the next, so a few thousand kilometers over land shouldn't be too much of a stretch.

Indeed, recent modeling efforts designed to predict where tick populations (infected or otherwise) are likely to spread in the coming years had to be tweaked in order to account for *Ixodes scapularis* ticks that have already been plucked off mammals in Newfoundland, an area beyond the accepted 425-kilometer limit. Either researchers are underestimating how far birds can fly during the length of time they're likely to carry infected nymphs or there are endemic populations much closer to Newfoundland that haven't yet been recorded.

One day we'll know the answer.

For now, this is what we know: Birds don't consult public health officials before they migrate. They don't file flight plans with researchers. They simply flap their way into regions where their hitchhiking passengers may never before have been seen. Those regions may have only recently warmed to the point where they're suitable for ticks to establish permanent populations. Or possibly they haven't hit that point yet. But that doesn't mean these regions can't play host to these hitchhiking ticks long enough for them to grab a meal from a large mammal before the cold weather sets in. These ticks may not make it through the winter, true enough, but that doesn't really matter if you're the large mammal they helped themselves to a meal from during their brief stay in your region.

The truth is, it's not just other people I don't recognize.

I don't recognize myself.

I spend more time looking in the mirror than a narcissist and yet it has nothing to do with being intoxicated by my looks. I'm baffled by the person I see looking back. There's a disturbing disconnect. I don't recognize the person I see in the mirror and yet the person I see in the mirror can only be me. That's a hard thing to come to terms with unless you're a character in a science fiction novel. In which case, it's Wednesday.

But I'm not a character in a science fiction novel. I didn't eat a poisoned apple. I didn't fall under the spell of an evil god. I didn't encounter a race of shape-shifting invaders.

No, wait. That's exactly what I encountered, but they're supposed to be changing their own characteristics, not mine. At no point were they supposed to steal my reflection. I mean, what's up with that? What purpose could it possibly serve Lyme to take away my ability to recognize myself in a mirror?

It's the eyes that bother me most. There's something odd about them. That's where wax figures fail to be convincing. Their creators don't get the eyes quite right and you can never truly capture the essence of a person if you don't master the eyes.

Which makes me wonder about my soul. Has Lyme done something truly sinister? Has it swapped out my soul and replaced it with one of its own design? That would certainly explain why my memory is so bad. You can't expect to remember things if your soul has been plucked from your body and replaced with that of an imposter.

Okay, that sounds loopy. My soul is fine. I just have to get used to the idea that I may never be able to see my own face again. I'm sure I'm not the first person this has ever happened to. Just because I've never heard of someone not being able to see her own face doesn't mean this sort of thing doesn't happen every day.

There are lots of things I've never heard of before.

I'd give you examples but, you know, that's a bit tricky.

ATTRACTING ATTENTION FROM AN UNUSUAL SOURCE

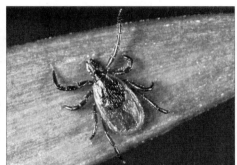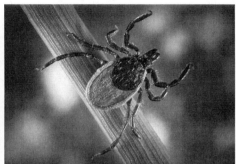

The black-legged ticks *Ixodes scapularis* and *Ixodes pacificus*

Although there are more than 850 species of ticks on this planet, we need only be concerned about the dozen or so that are capable of transmitting diseases to humans in North America. The two species standing proudly at the top of the most unwanted list when discussing Lyme disease are, of course, *Ixodes scapularis* and *Ixodes pacificus*.

I've included pictures of both of these ticks so that you could get a rough idea what your potential adversaries look like although, in retrospect, I'm not sure these pictures will be all that helpful to you. They aren't in the least bit helpful to me.

You see, for creatures that inspire such terrible infirmity in humans, these ticks are much smaller than you might think. The nymphal stage — the stage most likely to pass a Bb infection on to humans — has variously been described as being approximately the size of a poppy seed, the head of a pin, a freckle, or even the period at the end of this sentence. Whatever analogy you choose to go with, it's clear we're talking about a creature so small you'd likely not notice it unless it was crawling across your eyeball.

Okay, so maybe I'm exaggerating, but only slightly.

These photographs are of little use to you unless you have access to a microscope and a couple of decent entomology textbooks and likely you don't, so forget the photos and take this bit of advice: If you ever spot a poppy seed crawling across any part of your anatomy, remove it before it comes to a halt in your groin or your armpit or behind your left ear.

You could save yourself a lot of suffering if you do.

If you leave the healthcare system in search of someone or something that promises to cure you of your disease, you'll surely find what you're looking for. The trick comes in determining whether there's a realistic chance that the promised cure will materialize or whether you're about to be taken for a ride by someone unscrupulous, delusional, or both.

There's a lot of information about Lyme disease on the Internet. Much of it is contradictory, confusing and very, very angry. Some of it is downright hysterical. Still, I manage to learn some interesting things from that whimsical bastion of medical knowledge and the main thing I learn is that there's more than one way to skin this cat called Lyme.

I explore different options. Ayurveda. Traditional Chinese Medicine. Classical Homeopathy. Home remedies. You name it, I've googled it. But it all seems so hopeless. I'm lost and I'm confused and the fatigue is swallowing me whole.

I don't want to have to explain this debacle of an illness to a total stranger. I don't have the energy or the wherewithal to do that. I'm not even sure I can speak English anymore. But I have to try something.

So I throw caution to the wind and I make a phone call.

"Who gave you this number?"

"Does it matter?"

"Are you with Health Canada?"

"No."

"Because if you're with Health Canada, you have to tell me. It's entrapment if you don't."

"Well, I'm not, so I don't have to tell you anything except that I need help and I need it now, so can we drop the paranoia?"

"This will have to be a cash transaction. I can't take a cheque."

"Cash is fine."

"You can't tell anyone where you got this from."

"I wasn't planning to."

"I'm serious. As soon as you hang up the phone you need to destroy my name and number. Do you understand what I'm saying? You never met me. I don't exist."

"I can't tell you how reassuring that is."

In truth, there was more than one number I could've called to get my hands on what I was trying to get my hands on. I chose to dial the number of a distributor located in this country who was evidently feeling a bit touchy about Health Canada for reasons I didn't bother to get defined.

I have my own problems. I really don't care about his.

It's not illegal to own the supplement, mind you. I don't mean to imply that. You can even mix up a batch in your self-made laboratory if you know how much of one chemical to combine with the other and you'll be pleased to know that you can get those instructions off the Internet along with directions for making a bomb or starting your very own revolution. You could have a real party.

This not-to-be-named-here supplement (really more of a chemical) has long been used to sterilize counters, disinfect water supplies, strip textiles, and/or bleach pulp and paper. Health Canada doesn't appear to get too excited about any of that.

So I'll go out on a very short limb and guess that what gets the ministry hot under the collar is people who claim that swallowing a chemical that's commonly used in industrial settings for industrial purposes will confer health benefits.

Or maybe that particular supplier had just lobbed some LSD into his cornflakes.

I don't bother investigating because I'm on a mission and missions have a nasty habit of getting derailed by inconvenient details.

And besides, desperation does funny things to the mind. It causes you to do things you wouldn't normally do, like turning a deaf ear on that voice in your head that's telling you to stop dead in your tracks before you do something really stupid.

But then I already did something really stupid. I trusted the healthcare system to take care of me when I became ill. Nothing I've done before or since then can possibly touch that.

Certainly not this.

Let me just say that I find it surprising to discover that a creature so tiny you need a microscope to see it properly can be just as complex as the mammal that's peering down the eyepiece.

Among other things, ticks possess simple digestive, reproductive, nervous, and cardiovascular systems. They don't possess blood (except when they're drinking yours) although they do possess a substance quite similar to it called hemolymph, which, like blood, conveys oxygen and nutrients throughout their tiny bodies. Some of these ticks also possess my dear friend Bb, which can and does live quite happily in the midguts of the ticks it infects. Bb can also be found in the reproductive, nervous and excretory systems, but regardless of wherever else it can be found in a tick's body, Bb is always present in the midgut. That's important because when one of these seeds/freckles/periods/pinheads attaches to a host — regardless of whether that host is a mouse, a deer, or you — Bb navigates from the tick's gut into its salivary glands, where it's injected into its new host.

Most of the time, anyway.

Bb doesn't have to rely on a single mode of transportation to move into a new host. It can also be expelled into the host's body directly from the tick's guts, which is a polite way of saying that the tick can essentially puke the Lyme infection into its victim.

Nice.

I'm not sure that's any more pleasant to contemplate than the saliva mode of entry, but then I'm not sure there's anything pleasant about ticks.

Granted, I'm not trying too hard to find any examples.

I'm sitting in the corner of my bedroom wondering what attaches the spirit to the body and how it knows when to sever that bond. It's not the first time I've wondered this, but now, in the early morning haze, the answer is suddenly important.

I'm just not sure who to ask. My brain is throwing blanks. There are no theologians within earshot. Maybe I'll ask the air.

Or possibly I should explain why the answer is suddenly so important.

Yesterday I was following the low stone wall around the perimeter of my perennial garden. My plan was to stumble around to the front of the garden and contemplate the weeds swamping my peonies, even if I didn't actually pull them. Midway along the wall, my spirit floated away from my body like a helium balloon that's slipped its tether. My body remained earthbound while my consciousness rose a dozen feet or so above where it should be.

I can't say I had any deep thoughts at that moment. I was dizzy and nauseous and more concerned with the practical problem of how to get my spirit back inside my body than with what it meant for it to have broken free. There didn't seem to be a tether connecting my mind to my body, so it's not like I could reel myself back in, and yet, happily, my body and spirit remained inseparable despite no longer sharing the same physical space.

That raises some serious questions. For instance:

What's stopping my spirit from floating off into the clouds?

Are there limits on how far it can go before the bond between it and my body irrevocably breaks?

What happens if that bond does break?

Do I die?

Does my spirit float around like a ghost while my body dies?

I don't remember how I got back into my body. There's a blank where there should be a memory. But that was yesterday.

As I said, I'm sitting in the corner of my bedroom, and I'm staring up at the rafters where a spider is marching around in a way that suggests it's hopelessly lost. I know how it feels. You see, strictly speaking, I'm not actually sitting in the corner of my bedroom. My spirit is in the corner where the chair normally is while my body is lying on the bed. So I guess my spirit being where the chair normally resides is what's got me thinking of myself as sitting in the corner although, in retrospect, my viewing angle is too low for me to be sitting in that chair.

Maybe I am the chair.

That wouldn't surprise me. I think Lyme has beaten surprise right out of me.

Anyway.

My spirit is currently in the corner of the room and my body is lying on the bed. I'm refusing to look at it. What if it moves? It's best not to think about that. Instead I focus on the lost spider, pretending I care if it ever finds its way to its destination.

Nothing in life has taught me how to deal with a situation like this. I haven't got a clue how to go about reconnecting with my body. I don't even recall how I detached from it. I suppose I just floated off like I did yesterday, sideways instead of upwards. Supposition is all I have. There is no memory.

There is no time. I have no idea how long I've been in this state.

I'm disoriented and clueless, and believe me, I know it.

You sometimes hear about people who claim they can leave their bodies any time they wish — astral projecting, I believe they call it — like it's no big deal to spend the day soul-surfing the Himalayas, then reconnecting with your body again in time for the nightly news.

Trust me, it's a big deal.

I try to float towards the bed and discover that, with effort, I'm able to make some headway, although the visuals start to wobble and distort like surveillance camera footage of an earthquake.

I stop and so does the wobbling.

It occurs to me that I might be dead.

I disown the thought. I would know if I was dead. There'd be angels or ancestors or ethereal music guiding my journey through this transitory plane.

There'd better bloody well be cake.

I feel like a whisper.

Like a collection of photons.

And somehow I have to figure out how to get back into my body. Or how to leave it altogether.

I don't know which to choose. I don't even know if I'm the one who gets to do the choosing.

I don't know anything except that I'm not where I should be.

And that's a scary thing to know.

Ticks are often portrayed as being the insect equivalent of vampires, but that's not a particularly accurate analogy since technically ticks don't suck blood and since, also technically, vampires don't really exist.

Instead of planting their fangs and sucking, ticks cut into their victims' skin until they hit a blood vessel and then wait patiently as blood pools in the divot that was created for exactly that purpose. The tick then leisurely sips this blood like a socialite sips a martini. Yet unlike that martini-sipping socialite (hopefully, anyway), the tick alternates between sipping blood and injecting saliva for as long as it can get away with it. If you fail to notice the attached tick, it can keep this up for several days before dropping off.

And not noticing an attached tick is a very real possibility.

When a tick cuts into your skin it injects a plethora of substances designed, among other things, to avoid detection. One of these substances has a numbing effect that ensures you don't feel a tick bite the way you do the bite of a mosquito or a spider.

You don't feel it at all.

Ticks also tend to attach to warm, moist, out-of-the-way places on your body such as your groin, armpit, or really any place on the body that's covered with hair. This makes it highly unlikely that you'll notice an attached tick by accident.

But hey, maybe you get lucky and catch wind of the tick despite its best efforts to be stealth.

This could be because it becomes so engorged with blood that you either catch sight of it or run your fingers over its bloated body. Or maybe your tick was a bit reckless and attached itself to the back of your hand or the tip of your nose. Or maybe, just maybe, you're one of those conscientious folks who actively hunts for embedded ticks after frolicking in nature.

Some people actually do this.

Even if you do notice an attached tick, it can be difficult to remove it without causing further complications. Ticks lock themselves in place with a cement-like substance that makes it next to impossible to knock one off after it's attached itself to you. If you panic and try to do just that, there's a good chance that the tick's head — which is firmly cemented into place — will remain embedded in your skin. If you try to burn the tick off with a match or smother it with petroleum jelly, it'll only burrow deeper into your flesh, compounding the problem. And if you try to pull it out with your fingers, you'll likely only succeed in forcing the tick to vomit the contents of its guts — including Bb, if present — into your body.

This is definitely not the result you're going for.

The only real way to get a tick out of your skin once it's cemented itself in is to firmly grip the head of the tick with a pair of sharp tweezers and yank it straight out, head and all. This is a difficult feat to accomplish when your hands are shaking, so it's often better to let someone who doesn't currently have a tick embedded in any part of his or her anatomy do the honors.

Someone is talking to me and in theory I'm listening, but mostly I'm zoning.

I'm too tired to figure out who anyone is today and the strangest feeling is cascading down from my brain.

There's a lull in the admittedly one-sided conversation.

Possibly the speaker is waiting for a response from me.

That's optimistic.

I've got no clue what response to give.

And besides, something inside me is shifting in the most alarming way. Something I can't describe. I feel so strange. Like a snake slipping its skin. And my left hand is tingling in the most extraordinary way.

Then suddenly I know something I didn't know a moment ago: This has all happened before. Everything I'm seeing. Everything I'm thinking. Everything the specter is saying.

I've already experienced this exact moment a thousand times. I'm experiencing all thousand of those times right now.

I try logic. I tell myself that for some reason my central and peripheral nervous systems are out of sync and that's giving me the sensation of colliding with a present that I've already lived a thousand times, when no such thing is happening.

Bull. It may actually be the case, but it's still bull.

My soul is telling me something different; something that resonates deep inside me. It's telling me that time has collapsed. Past, present and future are occurring simultaneously. And nothing, not one single thing, will ever be unfamiliar to me again.

What else can I tell you about ticks?

Ixodes ticks have hard shells that make them resistant to dehydration, an important consideration for any creature that tends to cling to a blade of grass or the low branch of a shrub for as long as it takes to snag a passing mammal.

Ticks also have excellent carbon dioxide sensors, so if a mammal, any mammal, approaches the blade of grass a questing tick happens to be clinging to, it has more than sufficient time to raise its barbed legs and snag the mammal as it passes.

Ticks also have adaptable pH levels and body temperatures, two things that Bb has learned to deftly exploit. When a tick feeds on a mammal, the incoming blood lowers the tick's natural pH level and raises its body temperature, changes that alert Bb that it's going to have to rapidly alter its genetic structure in preparation for survival in the new host's environment.

This is where Bb's genius at antigenic variation really gets a chance to shine.

The bacterium analyzes the incoming blood on the fly and calculates what alterations need to be made to its genetic structure in order to optimize its chances of survival in its new host. It then promptly starts making those changes.

Now that's a neat bit of engineering. That would be like me preparing to morph into a mermaid the minute I dip my toe in an ocean. How cool would that be?

I'm implying, of course, that Bb can instantly change its structure like a mermaid on some magical beach. In reality, it takes time for Bb to alter its structure enough to ensure its survival in a new host, so the longer the tick remains attached to your body, the better the chances that a viable Bb infection will take hold.

How long?

Researchers have long claimed that a tick must remain attached to its host for between one and three days for Bb to have enough time to alter its DNA to the point where it's viable in a human body. However, there are recorded cases of Bb entering the central nervous system of its victims within a few hours of a tick attaching, which seems to suggest that at least some of the bacteria are able to do the Houdini thing much quicker.

Possibly a few hours. Possibly less than that. No one really knows for certain how long it takes for Bb to alter its genetic structure enough for at least one spirochete to be viable in a new host and it may be different depending on the type of tick, the type of mammal, the strain of Bb, the species of borrelia (if not Bb) and God knows what else. So, the sooner the tick is removed, the less likely that viable bacteria will be passed on.

That's really about all anyone can say on the subject.

It's midnight and the light from the wood stove is flickering against the ceiling. I have to look beyond the fluttering amber to see the vampire bat that's clinging to the shady side of the rafter. Its wings are spread wide as it waits for the perfect moment to swoop down and suck the tainted blood from my neck. That perfect moment will come when I close my eyes.

So I don't close my eyes. Instead I stare at this elusive, hunting bat. I can't make out its fangs or its eyes or even the veins branching out across its fragile wings, although I know instinctively that all those things are there. No, the only thing I can make out clearly is a shadow on the ceiling beyond the flickering light; a shadow that my brain has decided is a vampire bat despite my best efforts to convince it that what I'm really seeing is nothing more than an absence of light.

And absences don't cling to rafters or swoop down on their victims. They don't do anything at all. That's what makes them absences.

If I wake my husband he'll assure me that there are no gigantic bats gripping the rafters. He may even turn on the light to show me a ceiling that's vacant except for several impressive cobwebs that someone is really going to have to sweep away one of these days.

His proof will change nothing. I already know the bat isn't really there and being confronted with proof of what I already know won't make the slightest bit of difference.

The problem isn't what I know. The problem is what I believe. And what I believe is that a vampire bat is clinging patiently to the ceiling, waiting to suck my body dry the second I fall asleep. No amount of evidence is going to dislodge this idea, just as no amount of proof will ever convince a zealot there is no God. Belief shines an indelible light.

So I lie awake in the middle of the night, protecting my blood, or my soul, or whatever else this bat craves, from eternal damnation.

This is slightly more interesting than watching the northern lights flicking their fiery ropes across the midnight sky and a whole lot more disturbing. Not that the northern lights are at play tonight, but if they were, I'd be ignoring them in favor of a bat that only half my brain believes exists.

And that half believes it absolutely.

The supplement arrives in the mail without any fanfare soon after I send cash to the person whose name and contact information I no longer have in my possession, as per the somewhat paranoid agreement I had to strike before its mysterious supplier agreed to complete the transaction.

It's in a dark green bottle with a simple black and white label. No skull. No crossbones. I double-check.

And yet despite the lack of any obvious labeling to indicate that I'm handling a poison, I must confess that I'm afraid of the contents of the bottle. My hand tingles whenever I pick it up. Then again, my hand tingles whenever I touch just about anything these days, so that's not really saying much.

I can't help wondering if I'm doing something suicidal. I wouldn't even consider knocking back bleach or scarfing down Drano, so then why in God's name am I contemplating ingesting a textile bleaching agent? I mean, I know why I'm contemplating it. I'm trapped. I'm like a kidnap victim in the trunk of a car and I feel compelled to do everything in my power to escape my present predicament regardless of the price I may ultimately pay for that attempt. That's what I tell myself, anyway.

But am I willing to pay for it with my life?

I hesitate before answering.

I hesitate instead of answering.

Clearly I need to put more thought into this.

I close my eyes and become aware that something is staring back at me from inside my own head. The creature is suggestively human and it's peering at me with the curiosity of a child who's just discovered a strange bird perching on a kitchen counter.

The creature isn't menacing.

It just shouldn't be where it so obviously is, unless, of course, I'm dreaming. But I'm not dreaming, I'm fully awake — that much I'm sure of — and nothing should be inside my head but my own thoughts.

I wonder what the creature wants.

I wonder what I've done to attract its attention. And why is it staring back at me with such unblinking inquisitiveness? It just hangs there in the space between my mind and the outside world, translucent and bewitching. I can see this hologram just as well with my eyes closed as I can with them open, only the sight is a little less disturbing when my eyes are closed.

At least then I can pretend that I'm dreaming.

What I can't do is shut the hologram out.

I've grown used to this creature appearing with little or no warning except for a peculiar sensation that seems to pervade my entire existence and I must admit that for better or worse I've started to think of it as a guardian of sorts.

Not quite an angel. More like one of those gargoyles that perch on the roofs of medieval buildings, scaring away evil spirits. My brain has developed a gargoyle. Who knows why?

This creature, whatever else it may be, is grotesque. It's deformed and it's ugly. It's the sort of creature normally only ever seen in dreamscapes, and yet, here it is in front of me, watching me flounder. I hesitate to call this gargoyle a hallucination even though I know that's what it is, and I wonder why I'm seeing it.

I don't mean medically. I'm not really curious whether this gargoyle is the result of a bad mix of brain chemicals, inflammation in a specific part of my brain, a lack of cerebral blood flow, or just flat-out insanity. What I'm curious about is whether Lyme is really a disease or if it's something else entirely; something that a protective gargoyle needs to watch unblinkingly for the first sign of a cataclysm.

Maybe that's why researchers can't seem to nail it down. They're thinking of Bb as an organism when it's something else entirely. Something far more sinister. Something not necessarily of this world.

I take a deep breath and label the gargoyle a friend.

And I do my best not to alert those around me to what I'm seeing.

Nothing good could come of that.

A SOUND AND ALL ITS ECHOES

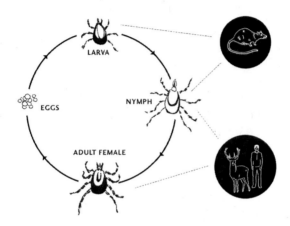

Let's talk some more about ticks.

Those ticks lucky enough to live full lives go through several transformations along the way; transformations which see them changing from eggs to larvae, larvae to nymphs and, finally, from nymphs to adults.

Now that's a lot of transforming.

So then it's hardly surprising that it can take up to two years for a black-legged tick to complete its journey from birth to death, assuming, of course, that it completes the full journey, which in the rough-and-tumble world of ticks is far from guaranteed. There are endless opportunities for them to croak along the way, but before they croak, these tiny arachnids participate in a life cycle that's fueled by blood.

That cycle begins in early spring when adult females lay their eggs. Sometime later that spring, or possibly even as late as early summer, those eggs hatch and from them crawl a fresh batch of larvae. In order for these larvae to transform into nymphs, they must drink the blood of whatever hapless rodent scuttles (or whatever bird hops) past. If that rodent or bird is infected with Bb, then any larvae feeding off it will contract the bacterium and carry it with them as they molt into nymphs during the coming autumn.

These nymphs must also drink blood, this time in order to make the transformation into adults. This blood meal again typically comes from a rodent or a bird, but it can also come from a human, if one happens to be around, and although the meal can occur during the autumn, it's more usual for ticks to put the feast off until the following spring or summer. Assuming, of course, that these nymphs make it through the winter, which is far from guaranteed. A whopping 90 percent of them will fail to complete the journey.

It should be noted that if any of these hungry nymphs were infected with Bb as a result of blood they drank when they were still larvae, the infection will now be transmitted to whomever or whatever they bite this time around. If, on the other hand, they managed to make it to the nymph stage without being infected, their infection-free status could abruptly change if they latch onto a mammal carrying the infection now. These newly infected nymphs will then join those that were infected as larvae in carrying Bb with them as they molt into adults, something that happens during the late summer or autumn of this second year.

This is when gender becomes important. Adult females must drink a mammal's blood, then find an adult male to mate with in order to lay their eggs. Adult males, however, exist solely to mate, then die. They rarely indulge in blood meals and therefore aren't likely to pass Bb on to humans or any other creatures. That crime lies with the females, whose blood meals come from large animals such as deer, dogs, or you.

This final feeding frenzy normally occurs during the autumn or early spring of the second year, but it can also occur during the winter if temperatures are mild enough for the ticks to become active, something that's a possibility whenever temperatures rise above 0C, which is happening increasingly on the coast and in the valleys of southern British Columbia as well as in other parts of southern Canada.

These adult females then go on to lay their eggs in the spring before dying.

That's about it.

Try as I might, I can never quite make the life cycle of a tick sound truly compelling.

A garbled stream of illogic spews from my lips and my husband looks baffled. We both try to figure out what I just said.

I'm not sure whether all the words I'm using are technically English and I'm not sure it matters.

With no rational thoughts framing their existence they hang in the air like exotic birds that may or may not be about to go for someone's eyes.

My husband abruptly leaves the kitchen.

His exit has nothing to do with my speech puzzles. No, it has to do with the phone that's ringing in his office and his rush to answer it before the client hangs up.

And that's a problem, since this conversation has been serving an important purpose.

Euphoria has been gaining in intensity for the past half hour and it's now hovering on the exquisite edge of agony. I've been trying to ignore it, suppress it, deny its right to exist. This was easier to do when I was talking to my husband. Focused thought seems to keep the euphoria in check, but the minute I stop — the minute my husband disappears from the kitchen — the euphoria transforms into a far more peculiar sensation centered somewhere around the middle of my brain.

What makes this sensation so peculiar is that I can't describe it, and it takes a lot for a writer not to be able to describe something, although mostly what it takes is the inability to locate any known thing that shares a characteristic with the odd sensation.

And I can't reference a single thing that feels like this. Nothing feels like this. I'm not even sure this feels like this.

The peculiar sensation rapidly reaches the point of overwhelming, like a tickling session that's gone on too long, and yet it's not entirely clear whether what I'm feeling is a physical sensation, a powerful new emotion, or a twisted hybrid of the two.

Foreboding rears its ugly head. Foreboding may be an understatement. End-of-the-world fear is more like it.

The peculiar sensation shoots upward. Then static radiates across my brain. My senses become increasingly vague and so do my thoughts. Everything seems so far away, so disconnected, as if I've been plunged into an aquarium and I'm watching the world from under water, behind glass, like a squid or a clam or a waterlogged sponge. I can't move, not even to blink.

Wait.

Wait.

Wait.

There's an eerie calm. Eerie because I feel calmer than I've ever felt in my life. I can move again, although I seem to be doing it in slow motion. My limbs feel waterlogged and so do my senses. Nausea is flooding down from my brain in waves and the left side of my body is rapidly losing strength.

My husband returns to the kitchen and stops short.

Surprise registers on his face.

"I wasn't expecting you to still be standing here."

I can't respond.

Not yet.

Several minutes pass before I'm able to speak, and when I do, the words come out slow and strangled and on the far end of intelligibility.

"How long were you gone?"

"Twenty minutes."

"That can't be true."

I would testify in court that my husband had only been gone a minute, but my husband disagrees. Somewhere between the peculiar sensation and the eerie calm, twenty minutes slipped away and I have no idea where they went.

A few weeks pass.

I think I'm safe.

But then the euphoria returns and brings with it the peculiar sensation, the burst of fear, the aquarium perception, the eerie calm, and the slow-motion reflexes that give way to nausea, vertigo, weakness and overwhelming fatigue. Often when the eerie calm arrives I'm standing (or sitting or lying) exactly where I was the last time I remember having a conscious thought, with no real sense that any time has passed.

And possibly no time has passed.

It takes something external to clue me in. My husband returning after twenty minutes on the phone is an excellent clue. So is glancing at a clock that seems to have leapt forward ten minutes in the blink of an eye.

The missing time is odd, confounding, but beyond being unsettling, it's also integratable. I just need to tell myself that time isn't really what our brains tell us it is. Our brains are imperfect filters. They tell us that time is linear and constant, when nothing could be further from the truth. The only constant in the universe is the speed of light.

Not time.

Never time.

It's just comforting for us to think that time moves at one rate, and always forward, despite any evidence to the contrary.

Like I said, the missing time episodes are integratable.

Other things aren't so easily integrated. Like when I'm standing in the living room and euphoria overwhelms me. My next conscious thought finds me standing in the bathroom at the far end of the loft, more than thirty feet from where I just was, with no memory of having traveled the distance and no passage of time in which to have accomplished the traveling. Imagine blinking and discovering that in the space of time it takes you to lower your lids and raise them you've been magically transported to the opposite end of your house.

It's all very *Bewitched.*

It's also very disorienting. I often don't recognize where I am even though I'm in a familiar place because my mind can't process the abrupt data splice. That's the awkward truth they never address on *Star Trek*, where the hero is simply beamed from the spaceship to the ruins of some ancient civilization on a previously uncharted planet and instantly has his bearings.

It probably helps that he knew the beaming was going to happen.

But still.

No matter how many times I'm transported, it always comes as a surprise. Sometimes I retrace the steps I must've taken to travel from the place I was an eye-blink ago to the place I so clearly am now, hoping to discover some evidence that will tell me what I was doing during the missing time span.

I mean, I must've been doing something.

I'm not quite ready to believe that a transporter beam was responsible for my abrupt relocation, so I must've traveled from point A to point B under my own steam.

There's something oddly compelling about these investigations.

The thought of what I might find electrifies the air around me.

Mostly I find nothing, but every once in a while I see where I set something down or left a door ajar or pushed a chair out of my way, and it's a bit like sensing the presence of a ghost.

My ghost.

But these investigations are rare. The curiosity is there, but so is the terrible sickness that floods the left side of my body, pulling me down and keeping me there for as long as it takes the worst of it to pass. Afterwards I wander around, sometimes for several days, with a brain that feels like it's packed in cotton, waiting for the sickness to finally pass and hoping with everything in me that time doesn't go missing again.

Until the next time it does.

White-footed mice are considered to be the primary source of blood meals for the larvae of *I. scapularis* ticks in Canada. If these larvae happen to be infected with Bb, then the mice they feed on will acquire it and carry the infection with them for the rest of their lives. Any tick that subsequently bites one of these mice becomes infected. That's not good news when you consider that the typical mouse lives and dies within 30 meters of where it was born, something that should clue you in to just how easily Lyme can become endemic to an area.

That's not to say that white-footed mice are the only source of blood meals for these larvae. Studies have shown that two species of shrew are also major hosts of Bb infections, and other rodents — chipmunks, squirrels, and wood rats among them — are no slouches either. Add into the mix the wide variety of songbirds that both the larvae and nymphs are more than happy to drink blood from and you have a whole lot of creatures that can and do keep Bb infections alive and kicking.

Chipmunks, squirrels, wood rats and shrews don't cover any more territory than mice do. Birds, on the other hand, travel long distances and some of them do this while carrying ticks that are doing their best to siphon off a little blood.

So look up. Way up.

Then look all around you.

We're literally surrounded.

Alfred Hitchcock would find this inspiring.

And yet Bb doesn't become entrenched in an area due solely to the presence of infected rodents and/or birds and the ticks that feed on them. No, in order for ticks to thrive in a region, there must be a healthy population of large mammals for the adult females to dine on. Enter your friendly neighborhood deer, which are easily hooked by the ticks that patiently cling to low-lying branches, brush, long grass, or whatever else happens to be low and handy as they await the opportunity to snag a host.

In truth, these ticks are just as happy to hook a dog or a human if there are no deer within striking distance. Cats, cows, goats, sheep, pigs, and chickens also make excellent targets. Indeed, the ticks that carry Bb have been known to attach themselves to literally hundreds of species of mammals, birds, and reptiles.

They are the very definition of indiscriminate feeders.

Bb can infect a surprising range of creatures to be sure, but not all of these creatures go on to develop the debilitating illness that we see in humans. Both deer and white-footed mice, for example, show no evidence of becoming ill from a Bb infection. It even appears that deer can rid themselves of the infection, meaning that not all deer infected with Bb go on to become permanent carriers of the bacterium. And then there are dogs, horses, and humans, all of whom can suffer varying degrees of infirmity from a Bb infection. In some cases, individual immune systems neutralize the infection with few or no symptoms ever surfacing, while in others, the illness becomes debilitating and can last for months or even years.

I wish I were a deer.

Or even a mouse.

Anything but what I actually am.

Sometimes in the middle of the night, I wake up to find myself lying on the foldout couch in my grandparents' den in a sleepy village not far from Niagara Falls. I breathe in the sickly sweet aroma of my grandfather's pipe that's resting on the desk against the opposite wall. Thick curtains muffle the early morning birdsong and domestic sounds echo down the hall from the kitchen at the far end of the bungalow.

Only I'm not in my grandparents' den.

I'm in my own bed in the open, airy loft of my log home in rural British Columbia. There are no tobacco scents or domestic sounds or muffling curtains here. The two places couldn't be more dissimilar, and yet, when the clock eases past midnight, thirty years melt away, depositing me in a place I haven't been since childhood.

Nothing is amiss.

Time has doubled back on itself and for a few misguided hours in the dead of night, the past becomes the present and an adult becomes a child.

Although *I. scapularis* and *I. pacificus* ticks are both known to carry and transmit Bb infections to humans and other mammals, researchers believe that a much higher percentage of *I. scapularis* ticks in endemic areas are infected with the bacterium than *I. pacificus* ticks. *I. scapularis* ticks are also reputed to be more eager to bite humans than their western counterparts are.

Those two pieces of information alone would seem to suggest that it's easier to contract Lyme disease in eastern Canada (where *I. scapularis* is dominant) than in British Columbia (where *I. pacificus* makes its home).

But such a suggestion ignores the geographical distribution of these tick species.

It seems *I. scapularis* has a fondness for hanging out in sparsely populated areas of its range, whereas the majority of infected *I. pacificus* ticks have a predilection for urban areas in southwestern British Columbia, where it's much more likely they'll come in contact with humans.

That's one way to even out the odds.

Or not.

There are other important differences between these two ticks that can impact infection rates. For instance, in its immature stages, *I. pacificus* favors lizard blood over mouse blood and some studies have shown lizard blood to be bactericidal, making it highly unlikely that any ticks subsequently feeding on that lizard will contract the bacterium.

Still, nothing can ever be simple when it comes to Lyme.

Although *I. pacificus* nymphs favor lizard blood, they've also been known to target wood rats, squirrels and birds, all of which have proven to be competent hosts for Bb, and the adults hanker for the blood of foxes, dogs, cattle, deer and, sadly, humans.

And there is no shortage of humans within its range.

The shaking is so violent I can't control my limbs. My arm shoots out, causing my fingers to strike the fold in the closet door. I'd move away if I could, but once the shaking starts I can't reposition my body.

I can't call out for help. I can't even cry. All I can do is rattle.

But it isn't as bad as it sounds. There's an overwhelming sense of euphoria when this happens. There's also a trance that keeps me from fully appreciating what's going on. As long as I don't strike a solid object, the whole experience can be quite pleasant, if a little disturbing.

When I do strike something, I often hit it so hard it leaves an impression. Literally. I'm amazed I haven't broken a finger or a foot, although I've managed to immobilize both for days at a time. And afterwards? Afterwards all I can remember is what I've written above. There's more to these shaking fits than what I've described, I'm certain of it, but the details are locked away in some compartment that my brain won't allow my curiosity to penetrate.

And if there's any mercy left in this wretched universe, it'll stay that way.

Now, if you're anything like me, you find yourself curious as to how researchers know that only a small percentage of *I. pacificus* ticks are infected with Bb.

Ticks aren't exactly the talkative type and, for as long as I've lived on my rural property in a Lyme-endemic region of British Columbia, I haven't once witnessed so much as a single researcher dragging flannel flags through the underbrush trying to catch any ticks — infected or otherwise — that might be lurking there. Yet researchers feel confident in stating that the chances of me coming in contact with an infected tick, even in an endemic area of the province, is quite low.

How do they know?

The primary method of keeping track of infected ticks in BC (and the rest of Canada) has long been passive surveillance, which essentially means that when a tick is removed from a human or an animal, it can be sent off to a government or university laboratory and, assuming that it's the right sort of tick and arrives at a qualified lab in a testable condition, it will then be tested for any evidence of Bb.

This method has been in place in Canada since 1990. There are definite pros and cons to it.

On the pro side of things, the rate of infection in ticks collected through passive surveillance tends to be higher than in ticks collected through active surveillance, a process which sees researchers physically going to areas in which Bb-infected ticks are suspected to reside and collecting both ticks and wild rodents to test for the presence of infection. And since the ticks collected through passive surveillance often come from regions other than those known to have endemic populations of infected ticks, a cluster of infected ticks arriving from a single location can alert researchers to potential new areas of concern.

Since passive surveillance has long been the primary basis for projections regarding tick populations and rates of infection in BC, it stands to reason that if the figures are skewed by the surveillance method being used then they're likely being skewed in a way that shows an elevated percentage of Bb infection in ticks. So when the figures are tabulated and it's subsequently reported that the percentage of infected ticks in British Columbia is low, that should be an accurate assessment.

But is it really?

Passive surveillance has several drawbacks.

First, the vast majority of ticks collected from humans and dogs are adult females. They're much easier for the average person to spot than nymph ticks, which are so tiny they're barely noticeable even if you happen to be looking for them. Adult females, on the other hand, are large enough that they're often spotted and removed. If that removal comes at the hands of a doctor, a veterinarian, a wildlife biologist, or some other concerned party, then sometimes that tick will make its way to a lab for testing.

But often it won't.

Seriously, who needs the paperwork?

Regardless, most Lyme infections in humans are the result of bites by those oh-so-hard-to-spot nymphs, and not the adult ticks that form the bulk of the ticks tested in this province. Rarely are these nymphs caught biting their victims and so passive surveillance tests ticks for possible Bb infection during a stage of their development other than the one most likely to spread the bacterium to humans.

Is that significant?

With each transformation, a tick must take a blood meal and with each blood meal an opportunity arrives for that tick to acquire a Bb infection that it subsequently carries for the rest of its life. This means that adult ticks should have the highest rates of infection of any phase in a tick's life cycle. So even though those hard-to-spot nymphs are more likely than an adult tick to bite a human, the adult tick must necessarily be the most infected stage of a tick's life. Therefore assessments of tick infection rates should, if anything, be elevated due to the reliance on passive surveillance (and therefore adult ticks).

There's a comforting logic to that argument.

It helps me to ignore the fact that the vast majority of nymphs don't make it to adulthood.

I'm not sure if that's important.

But it's knowledge that lingers.

While researching passive surveillance, I stumble across a fly in the statistical ointment. It comes in the form of a 2008 interview with an official from the British Columbia Centre for Disease Control who stated that over a period of ten years, 10,000 ticks were collected from humans and animals in BC and sent in to be tested for the presence of Bb. Based on the results of those tests, the agency felt confident in announcing that the incidence of Bb infection in ticks in this province is very low.

I do the math.

Ten thousand ticks tested over ten years works out to, on average, 1,000 ticks per year being tested in a province of just under a million square kilometers.

That's one tick for every 100 square kilometers.

That's nothing.

Or rather, nothing would be better, because if no ticks had ever been tested, then public health officials wouldn't feel so confident in stating that Bb infection rates of ticks in this province are low. Even if all thousand of those annual ticks had been collected from known Lyme hot spots in the province, they would give us only a narrow window on the situation in limited areas. However, it's more likely that those ticks came from multiple locations across the diverse geography of this province, something that can only dilute the data.

As it stands, the number of ticks being tested is so miniscule that any comfort I initially derived from the use of the passive surveillance for keeping tabs on the Bb infection rates in this province was immediately erased.

There simply isn't enough data to support those claims. Or, at least, there isn't enough data to satisfy me that those claims can be supported.

When attempting to construct an accurate picture of the chances of a human contracting a Bb infection in the province or even in the country, testing ticks during the nymph stage of their life cycle — when they're most likely to pass on the infection to humans — would certainly be helpful.

It would eliminate an important variable.

However, in order to get their hands on those nymphs, researchers would need to engage in active surveillance, collecting significant numbers of ticks from target regions as a part of well-designed studies, something that would require an increase in the number of research dollars devoted to advancing our collective understanding of tick-borne illnesses. After all, actively sending researchers out into the field adds a layer of expense to surveillance activities that doesn't exist when ticks are voluntarily turned in. It also adds a greater number of ticks into the census and allows researchers to target specific regions, species, and life-cycle stages, all of which would lend greater accuracy to statements about geographic distribution and risk.

In recent years, efforts have been made to conduct active surveillance on a limited basis and information derived from those activities is starting to trickle in, albeit on a somewhat piecemeal basis. Active surveillance in British Columbia has shown that the distribution of *I. pacificus* ticks is widespread across much of southern BC. It has also shown that Bb is present in nature (in ticks and in rodents) at several locations. The relatively modest numbers of infected ticks discovered at these locations, along with the presumed disinclination of *I. pacificus* to feed on humans, has prompted health authorities to conclude that the risk of human infection is much lower in BC than in eastern Canada.

Still, these were limited surveys covering very little territory and undertaken infrequently.

They're a start, but only a start.

In time, these and other studies will no doubt give us a more complete picture regarding the risk of exposure to infected ticks in British Columbia.

Sooner would be preferable to later.

But I don't know how to speed time up.

I only know how to slow it down.

Memories are missing. Big ones. I'm confused by the loss and fumbling for possible explanations.

What makes these memory gaps so discombobulating is that I often don't know a memory is gone until someone starts to reminisce about some event or place or person we have in common and I can't access a single memory associated with that reminiscence. Nothing resonates.

From my perspective, the event never occurred; the place was never visited; the person never known. But then I'll stumble across a photograph of myself in front of a monument, find a souvenir amongst my keepsakes, or encounter some other random bit of evidence to tell me that I don't have a complete picture of what's gone down in my life.

It's the photographs that bother me the most. I have no emotional connection to them. Not even a hint of memory. Yet here's a picture of me enjoying myself in a place I'd swear I've never been and I put that photo in an album as if it's important to me. Why is it important? I wish I knew.

There are times when a memory hovers like a ghost on the horizon. I get the sense that if I could only try a little harder, if I could only get one more synapse to fire, then this ghostly memory will explode into view. But the effort to remember causes nausea and fatigue to sweep down from my brain, forcing me to lie down before I vomit or pass out or both.

Sometimes I wonder what the point of being alive is. If I'm not going to remember my past then what's the point of having one? Or a present, for that matter, if it's going to be whimsically erased within seconds of occurring.

I wish I could remember what I was thinking or doing a minute ago, but it's hidden behind a rubbery membrane that I can't quite push through. So I ask — because who wouldn't ask at this juncture — will the person I am tomorrow be the result of accumulated life experiences I cannot remember?

What really irritates me about Lyme punching holes in my memory is that there's no rhyme or reason to what gets hit.

My wedding? Gone.

Perching on a wall in front of Yosemite's famous Half Dome? Not there.

Graduating from university? Nope.

Riding a bicycle around Pelee Island while butterflies erupt around me? Nice try.

Thank God for photographs and other people's memories. They may be disorienting — they may seem like evidence being presented at a trial — but they're all I have to tell me that many events ever took place.

And for that I'm grateful.

Had I known I was going to lose so much, I would've taken more photographs.

Yes, my memory sucks, but here's something I do remember: There's a dark green bottle with a black and white label — no skull, no crossbones — loitering in the cupboard behind a motley collection of spices. I see it peering over the tops of smaller, less intimidating bottles every time I pop open the cupboard door.

It taunts me.

It tempts me.

Every once in a while, I take the bottle out of the cupboard. Sometimes I roll it between the palms of my hands. At other times I examine its label although, in truth, I long ago memorized its instructions. I could whip up a batch of this miracle supplement (that claims to cure everything from malaria to HIV) any time I want, then knock it back like whiskey in a Wild West saloon. I just can't seem to bring myself to do it and I find myself wondering just what it'll take to tip the scales.

Just how much deeper into this abyss must I sink before I do something drastic?

The answer comes sooner than I expect.

RAIN ON A DISTANT ROOF

Those awful, homicidal fevers return without warning. They arrive at dusk and burn like signal fires throughout the night. I don't know who — or what — they're signaling and it's probably better not to ask. It's probably better not to even wonder.

It's just that I need a distraction from the pain shooting from my spine and pointless conjecture gives me that. Lyme is in a diabolical mood tonight. It's affixed clamps to every single vertebra in my spine and is twisting them all in very different directions. Lightning forks out, striking my fingers and teeth and the backs of my eyes.

My ribcage feels like someone has taken a nail gun to it. Repeatedly. Abstractly. Then set it on fire. Breathing only fans the flames, so I try to suck oxygen in through the pores of my skin. It doesn't work. I don't know why I thought it would.

The pain candles, scattering sparks across the surface of my body.

My skin is alive. My skin is on fire. Soon it will scorch the sky.

I'm in desperate need of a distraction.

I envision lava gushing from the heart of a shattered mountain.

Not helpful.

I try to name the swirling gases that fuel the sun's corona.

Even worse.

I imagine conveyor belts vibrating with glass and tacks and the fangs of vipers.

Clearly I'm not getting the hang of this.

I contort my body, trying to find a position — any position — that will pop the clamps. But Lyme is in no mood for mercy tonight.

Standing can only make the situation worse, but I do it anyway, hoping to stagger as far as the bathroom so that I can run warm water into the bathtub and soak the pain away.

My plan is to drown lightning in water.

My plan is a bad one.

The second my spine hits the heat it buzzes like a tube crammed full of tiny, frantic bees. I consider stabbing a syringe into the heart of the tumult and pulling up on the plunger until each and every one of those bees has been extracted. But I don't have a syringe and, considering what I'm contemplating doing with one, that's probably a good thing.

So I float in the slowly cooling liquid, fixating on the bees that are stinging the walls of their long, narrow, oddly contorted prison. My hope is that their venom will somehow counteract the pain.

I'm doing more than hoping.

I'm listening to the rub of my foot against the end of the tub. And there's another sound — like bloated raindrops bursting against a distant metal roof — and I'm wondering which part of my anatomy is capable of generating this soundscape.

Maybe the bees are imploding.

Then again, maybe it's the cysts that are imploding, spewing vulnerable twizzles of yarn into the open where my immune system has a snowball's chance in hell of recognizing them for what they are and launching an attack. Or maybe it'll attack my spinal cord instead.

My immune system is a psychopath.

And it's a psychopath that's going to lose this battle against a foe that has turned out to be so much stronger and more creative than I ever could have imagined. When the first fevers struck all those months ago, I had everything a person needs to successfully fight them off — energy, stamina, the belief that I would ultimately prevail — but with each recurrence I lost a little bit more of each of those things and wasn't able to regain them when the fevers finally left me. Instead I've slowly and progressively grown weaker, more fatigued, less certain that there's a future in my future.

The one thing I've known all along is that my only chance for survival is for those rollicking fevers to leave and never return. And they had.

Until now.

It's hard to survive a fever that tops 42C. Look that up if you don't believe me. And yet that's just what my body needs me to do with no fuel left in the tank. There's no reason to believe that I'll make it through the night.

So I listen to the bloated, bursting raindrops and try to convince myself that the spinal bees are under my command, ready, willing, and able to sting those malevolent spirals the second they burst from their protective cysts and encounter an army the likes of which they never imagined would be raised against them.

Then no more spirals.

Hallelujah.

I come to, still in the tub.

I hadn't realized I was going to pass out, but there you go.

I try to take charge of my thoughts; only they keep drifting back to that non-existent syringe.

It's a distraction and one that keeps me from thinking about the terrible sickness that's flooding down from the base of my skull. Part nausea, part agony, part hypnotic, it makes me feel like smoke billowing across an uninhabited valley.

What would happen if I were to use my fantasy syringe to puncture an artery? Would blood stream out in a perfect red jet and swirl the water pink? It's hard for me to picture my blood as anything other than thick and black as tar, so maybe the water would instead turn dark and cloudy like an aquarium filled with octopus ink.

Weakness floods down my left arm.

I stop thinking about the octopus ink and start thinking about the brilliant white light that greets me whenever I close my eyes. Maybe instead of blood, light will come streaming out of the needle hole with laser-like intensity. And maybe, just maybe, I'll get lucky and when the light hits the water it'll short-circuit what's left of my tick-shattered life.

It amuses me to think that if I were to stab a needle into an artery I'd die of electrocution.

The thought is calming.

I have no idea why.

The humming sensation is leaking from my spine and saturating my skin, turning millions of innocent cells into electrocytes. If a fly were to collide with my shoulder right now, it would sizzle. then disappear in a tiny puff of smoke.

I hold tight to that thought. I have to. It's the only thing between me and the horrible pressure at the base of my skull. It feels very much like someone is trying to force a baseball up into my brain and isn't about to let my skull stand in his way. Maybe it's a huge ball of blood with no place to go.

Where is that syringe?

Too late. Nausea has hit the boiling point. I slither from the tub and crumple on the bathmat with my cheek pressed against the cold tile floor. I hope against hope that the nausea will soon pass or at least scale down a notch.

Not tonight.

The baseball breaches my skull and the vomiting begins. And once the vomiting begins, nothing can stop it.

PART 3: PARADISO

*"Transhumanize" — it cannot be explained
per verba, so let this example serve
until God's grace grants the experience.*

— Dante Alighieri
Paradiso

THE MAGIC HEALTH FAIRY

It's the distinctive chainsaw buzzing of her wings that alerts me to the Magic Health Fairy's presence. She doesn't deign to arrive through an open window or a sloppily closed door like some lowly mosquito. No, she wriggles through a crack in the log wall, her wings doing the cussing instead of her mouth.

Her mouth is meant for more delicate matters.

I know I'm in trouble when that nasty fairy perches on my shoulder and starts whispering in my ear. I have no idea what she's saying since, as usual, she insists on delivering her message in a mutilated form of Spanish.

Whatever it is, it seems to be urgent.

So I listen to the hisses and the pops and the musical delivery, trying to pick out individual words.

Nothing comes.

I wish she'd just get away from me.

The Magic Health Fairy pinches my ear. She can read my mind even though my mind is speaking English. This is how I know she's capable of delivering her message in a language I can understand if she really wants to.

But she doesn't really want to.

She wants me to guess.

She wants me to make mistakes.

It's the suffering that attracts the fairy more than the illness.

The Magic Health Fairy looks like what I imagine Tinkerbell might if she'd downed a dozen shooters and set fire to her hair. Through some existential blunder she's been charged with helping the desperately ill in cold, dreary Canada when she'd much rather be living it up in Monte Carlo.

Her every gesture conveys disgust.

Yet despite her miserable attitude, the Magic Health Fairy does her duty, wriggling into the room and whispering in my ear, albeit incomprehensibly. I suspect she's following her orders to the letter by bringing me the message at all. The letter, however, clearly failed to specify that the message must be delivered in a language its recipient can understand.

I wonder if she has a medical degree.

I wonder if she has a boyfriend.

The Magic Health Fairy has many skills beyond stubbornly bringing me messages I can't interpret. She sprinkles stardust in my eyes and kicks my heart until it jumps. She pulls on my nerves so hard that lightning strikes my ribs and eyes and fingers. And while she does all this I try to determine whether she believes herself to be helping or whether she's merely working out some rage.

My money's on the rage.

Still, I've learned a few things about the Magic Health Fairy despite her attempts to remain opaque. For instance, I've learned that just because she has wings, that doesn't make her an angel.

This is one tough little fairy.

Her tiny wings are ripped and riddled with holes that appear to have been repaired with the silk from spider webs. This should make it impossible for her to fly. Maybe she can't and that's why she's doing time with me when she could be assisting malaria victims in Africa.

But I'm no angel either and I don't care why she's here as long as she makes herself useful. So I loop some dental floss around her ankle and attach her to my radio's antenna. Sparks shoot from her ears and her wings buzz so fast they sound like miniature weed-whackers set on high.

This isn't torture for torture's sake.

No, there's a payoff, at least for me.

Hitched to my radio, the Magic Health Fairy brings in stations from Japan and Russia and who knows where else. The words sound like pictographs, so I try to see them with my ears. Some of the languages are so strange I swear my fairy-amplified radio is catching chatter from a neighboring galaxy. Judging by the look on the fairy's fury-scorched face, she thinks so too.

I turn away from her and train my attention on the unfamiliar number registering on my thermometer. I wonder just how high a fever can go before one's brain starts to smell like pot roast.

The Magic Healthy Fairy flexes her tattered wings.

Without saying a word, she indicates that my fever has reached the upper limits of survivability.

That sends a chill down my spine.

The fairy once again starts to speak, in Spanish, with increasing intensity, and even though I have no idea what she's saying I know she's once again delivering her message without breaking her own stubborn code. As I listen to its incomprehensible contents I find myself wondering who is sending me this message and why in God's name she or he would entrust it to a partially mangled fairy.

That does it.

I'm going to send a message back.

It will definitely be in English and it'll be so rude there'll have to be consequences.

Those consequences are what I'm after.

I need this to end.

I can't end it myself.

So I need the fairy's help.

And that's a desperate thing to need.

My brain feels blistered and breath is rasping through my lungs, but I've made it through the night and that's all that really matters.

Or maybe it doesn't matter anymore.

My neck is strangely silver and my face looks like it's been dipped in bleach.

And my heart is beating in loops.

It feels as if some joker has parked an anvil on my chest. With each breath it settles just a little bit lower and I fight to draw air into lungs that are slowly being crushed, only the harder I battle, the less satisfying the results. It would be easier to stop breathing altogether than to fight against suffocation.

I fight anyway.

Some small part of me refuses to give up.

I try to sit up, but everything spins then turns black. When I come to, I roll onto my side and lie still, fighting off the spins and the blackness until I find the strength to get out of bed. But my legs buckle and I land on my knees with my shoulder against the wall. I try to catch my breath and my equilibrium. There's no feeling below my knees so I'm going to have to crawl if I want to get anywhere, but that's proving difficult. Every time I get into position, lightning bolts shoot down my spine and into my left arm.

Strange, rubbery lightning bolts.

So I don't have a whole lot of choice but to crawl, using only my right arm, which is even more pathetic than it sounds. I stop and hug the floor too many times to count, each time waiting for the nausea and the dizziness and the gasping to pass. And I try to ignore the terrible cracking pains fanning out across my chest and the rapidly worsening tremor in my left arm.

My heart is still beating in loops, only now it's started skipping the odd one like a novice learning how to knit. I should probably stop what I'm doing. I should probably lie flat on my back on the hardwood floor and wait for all of this to pass, but I'm tired of lying on the floor. I've been doing that for endless months now and where has it gotten me?

Here. And here is pretty messed up.

Also, there's an imperative at play. A now-or-never feeling.

So I crawl. I go down the stairs on my backside, then it's back to my knees. It takes far too long to drag myself to the kitchen, but I do it, and when there I manage to hoist myself onto my feet on the fourth try and grab the green bottle from the cupboard, knocking over several spice bottles in the process.

The textile bleaching agent.

I know how to mix up a batch.

I've known that for a while.

I've just never had the nerve.

Until today.

So I do the mixing.

Then I do the drinking.

Salvation or suicide remains to be seen. But one way or another, I'm counting on it to bring this whole hellish adventure to an end.

TOXIC MYTHS

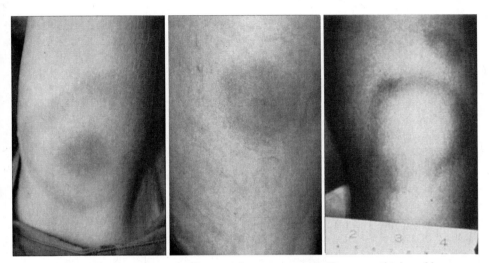

Erythema migrans rashes —bull's-eye rash on arm, non-bull's-eye on thigh and knee

There is no consensus on how to diagnose Lyme disease if a patient doesn't have a distinctive EM (erythema migrans) rash and — depending on which source you consult — the percentage of patients who develop such a rash can be as low as 20 percent. The percentage who develop the bull's-eye rash so definitive of Lyme is less than 10 percent and a significant number of Lyme patients who present with neurological symptoms don't recall ever having seen a distinctive rash on their bodies at any point during their illness.

And yet.

Emphatic statements by some Canadian public health officials that 80 percent of Lyme sufferers in this country develop an EM rash are difficult to justify unless, of course, those statements are based on research from that other, more populous, country to the south, and rubber-stamped into the knowledge base here.

A great many Lyme sufferers in this country, myself included, have never seen an EM rash anywhere except in medical journals. And, fascinating though that rash truly is, it's hard to connect it to the illness I'm suffering from, making statements by public health officials seem a little abstract.

I often wonder how well they really know the disease.

I'm guessing not well.

In response to some rather pointed criticism directed at an article on Lyme disease published by public health officials from British Columbia in 2011, the article's authors claimed not to be familiar with the details of any patient's struggle with Lyme disease.

I believe them.

If you'd asked me, I would've told you that I don't honestly believe public health officials in this province have any direct experience with Lyme disease patients. Their worlds are filled with theoretical patients, not flesh-and-blood ones.

Flesh-and-blood patients are messy, unruly, hard to constrain. Theoretical patients dance like marionettes on the end of hypothetical strings.

It's these theoretical patients that public health officials speak of when they discuss Lyme disease in articles and in sound bites on television.

In one article whose intended audience was medical doctors, the only symptom of early Lyme disease that health officials list is a distinctive erythema migrans (EM) rash that spreads out from a tick bite until it exceeds five centimeters in diameter. The rash may or may not have a central clearing. It may or may not look like a bull's eye.

That public health officials often spend more time on this rash than any other symptom of Lyme when trying to educate doctors about the disease should give you an idea of the importance they place on this single diagnostic symptom.

Dear doctors: Forget everything else; just look for the rash.

Officials do normally acknowledge that the initial phase can also give rise to flu-like symptoms, including fatigue, headaches, muscle and joint pain, swollen lymph nodes and fevers, but not nearly with the degree of emphasis they place on the rashes.

It's a bit unsettling.

The true percentage of Lyme sufferers who develop such a rash has yet to be determined and is complicated by the fact that the true number of people who suffer from Lyme disease in Canada is unknown and will likely remain so until accurate testing is developed, doctors are better trained to clinically diagnose the illness, public health officials find better ways of enumerating the infected, and toxic myths about the illness fade from public discourse.

Those halcyon days are still a long way off.

This leaves Lyme disease sufferers caught in the crossfire of a medical debate we had no part in creating except for the fact that we exist when public health officials would prefer that we didn't.

We are a problem. A blight on the diagnostic landscape. A mistake in need of correction.

It's a difficult situation, and all this emphasis on rashes only makes matters worse.

I know why they do it, of course. The alternative is to admit openly and publicly that in the absence of a distinctive rash there is no defining symptom for a Lyme infection and in admitting that they leave themselves open to widespread public hysteria. After all, no one can actually say you don't have Lyme disease unless strictures — arbitrary though they may be — are placed on who qualifies as having the illness and who doesn't.

So hope that if you're ever bitten by a tick you:

a) remember the tick bite;

b) have the good sense to be bitten in a known endemic area;

c) have the even better sense to acquire the infection in spring or early summer; and

d) develop an expanding rash (possibly bull's-eye, possibly not) that's at least five centimeters in diameter.

Do all of that and you'll be in the minority.

You'll be a medical cliché.

But you'll also stand a decent chance of being diagnosed with Lyme disease unless, of course, you get one of those doctors who mistakes your rash for a spider bite or an infected mosquito bite and then you'll be back in the same boat with the rest of us.

Sorry the ride was so short.

Turn up with any symptom other than a rash — or worse — turn up with some oddball collection of symptoms and Lyme will likely not be considered until things have progressed beyond the point where the few weeks of antibiotics you're likely to be prescribed will have a snowball's chance of curing it.

It's certainly a conundrum. But then why wouldn't it be? Lyme is a master of deceit. Its symptoms can be subtle, non-specific, and easily assigned to more common ailments. More often than not, that's exactly what happens.

The high degree of variability, diversity, and severity of symptoms means that a significant number of Canadians who are eventually diagnosed with Lyme were initially misdiagnosed with anything from chronic fatigue syndrome to bipolar disorder to amyotrophic lateral sclerosis (aka ALS or Lou Gehrig's disease) and just about everything in between. That's because once Lyme disease progresses beyond the first stage, sufferers report wide-ranging symptoms affecting the circulatory, digestive, excretory, musculoskeletal, nervous, reproductive and respiratory systems.

That's a lot of systems.

It's also a lot of symptoms. They include (but are by no means limited to) abnormal heart rhythms, bone pain, confusion, dental problems, diarrhea, disorientation, dizziness, extreme fatigue, facial weakness or paralysis, flashing lights, light sensitivity, headaches, impaired speech, insomnia, joint pain, memory loss, migraines, mood swings, numbness, panic attacks, paralysis, rashes, seizures, sexual dysfunction, shortness of breath, sudden deafness, tingling sensations, twitching muscles, unexplained weight gain (or loss), and weakness. And that's the short list.

Our dear friend Lyme is a chameleon. A doppelgänger without compare. Its symptoms overlap with a breathtaking number of diseases. Those illnesses include Alzheimer's disease, anxiety, colitis, Crohn's disease, depression, encephalitis, fibromyalgia, irritable bowel syndrome, lupus erythematosus, Meniere's syndrome, mononucleosis, multiple sclerosis, obsessive-compulsive disorder (OCD), Parkinson's disease, prostatitis, Raynaud's phenomenon, rheumatoid arthritis, schizophrenia, scleroderma...and the list goes on and on and endlessly on.

Some Lyme sufferers get off easier than others. For them, the symptoms are limited to arthritis, depression, or anxiety. For others the illness has a severe impact on brain function, interfering with neurotransmitters, damaging synaptic connections, causing brain atrophy, cerebral volume loss, and neuronal death. The areas of the brain hardest hit by Lyme include the hippocampus, the striatum, the limbic cortex, the neocortex, and the amygdala. Disruptions in these areas can cause, among other things, problems with memory and recall, confusion, motor co-ordination deficits, emotional and behavioral disorders as well as impairments to language skills, conscious thought, and spatial reasoning.

Bb also suppresses the immune system and alters vital processes.

It hijacks hormones, proteins and inflammatory chemicals.

It can enter each and every cell in the body and can inflame the brain, nerves, heart, blood vessels, joints and connective tissues. It can also cause dysfunction in the hypothalamic-pituitary-adrenal (HPA) axis, resulting in imbalances in any number of hormones, including thyroid and fertility, DHEA, leptin and many others that you've likely never heard of.

The result is sheer chaos.

Modern medicine still doesn't know the full range of symptoms that Bb is capable of causing. In fact, researchers haven't even nailed down how or why Bb causes illness when it enters the human body.

They just know that it does.

What is known is that Lyme sufferers are reporting wide-ranging symptoms that impact every conceivable area of the body, with many reporting symptoms not traditionally associated with the disease. And far too little research has gone into determining why.

So then, where are these atypical symptoms coming from?

Are they the result of co-infections with other organisms?

Novel strains of the Bb bacteria?

Other species of borrelia?

Antigenic variation?

Individual immune response?

Any or all of the above?

No one has the definitive answer. Hypotheses abound. Or should I say guesses?

And the answers will one day arrive. Just not yet. Our time hasn't arrived.

It's the waiting that's killing us. Slowly. Painfully. Bit by bit.

Bb, with its awesome powers of transformation, becomes exponentially more difficult to eradicate the longer it stays in the body, resulting in a chronic infection that can takes months and sometimes years of adequate treatment to cure.

Assuming it's even curable. There's considerable debate over whether a Lyme infection that's gone untreated for more than a month can be cured using the treatment options available today. Maybe not.

But we have to try. We have no choice. The suffering is inhumane.

A cure might not be possible. True enough. In order to cure Lyme, you'd have to annihilate every one of Bb's survival forms: every cyst, every biofilm, every cell-wall deficient rebel. The failure to eliminate a single organism could allow Bb to regenerate and eventually you'll feel the effects.

Maybe not this week. Maybe not even this year. But eventually it'll return like a psychotic ex-lover who just can't get enough of you.

So remission may be a better target than an all-out cure.

Lyme can go latent in any one of its three stages. If you play your cards right, the symptoms can one day just up and disappear, regardless of whether the illness is technically cured or not, and those symptoms may not return for a very long time. Just don't ask me which cards to play.

And try not to think too much about the negative side of this equation. That negative side being that when someone suffering from Lyme walks into a doctor's office without a rash and with non-specific symptoms, they'll likely leave under the impression that the problem, whatever it is, will go away on its own.

And it will appear to.

Then weeks, months, years, maybe even decades later, that same unfortunate someone will develop a different set of symptoms — symptoms which are not related back to the original problem — and Lyme will likely once again fail to be recognized.

Medical ignorance shapes the lives of Lyme sufferers like nothing else. Many doctors don't even know when to suspect a Lyme infection. They persist in believing it's a rare illness. There are even those who staunchly claim that Lyme doesn't exist in this country despite a mountain of evidence to the contrary.

It's the patients who bear the brunt of those misguided beliefs.

A disease that knows not to cross an invisible line on a map is indeed an awesome thing, if indeed that's what happening. Serious questions have been raised about the alarming number of people being diagnosed with MS in this country; the fear being that many people in Canada who are living with advanced Lyme infections are being told that they have an incurable autoimmune illness instead.

The symptoms of the two illnesses often overlap.

Both are known to cause white matter lesions.

Both are suspected to cause chronic cerebro-spinal venous insufficiency (CCSVI), a condition which prevents blood from efficiently returning to the heart from the brain.

And both can cripple.

Of all the illnesses that advanced Lyme disease gets mistaken for, MS tops the list. Many of us who end up being diagnosed with Lyme have sat in doctors' offices or hospital beds listening to doctors making the case for why they think MS may be the cause of our symptoms.

Those conversations leave an indelible impression.

Knowing what I know now, I wouldn't accept an MS diagnosis without doing everything in my power to first rule out Lyme.

With or without the help of doctors.

It concerns me how many times I heard doctors mention MS back in 2007 and how easily I became convinced that it would ultimately get the blame for my illness. But for the efforts of one doctor seeking to rule out Lyme disease as the possible cause for the sudden, dramatic decline in my health, an MS misdiagnosis may very well have been my fate.

Maybe that makes me a lucky person after all.

However, I'm more inclined to believe that God is having a pretty good laugh at my expense.

The textile-bleaching agent that I drank in an effort to rid myself of Lyme turned out to be surprisingly effective. It didn't cure me of the illness — so far nothing has accomplished that feat — but it did knock the symptoms back far enough to convince me that Lyme could be adequately treated by something other than pharmaceutical antibiotics.

In that respect, it was a true gateway drug.

I probably should mention that in 2010, Health Canada issued an official advisory warning Canadians not to ingest the textile-bleaching agent that I've referred to in this book and implicated it in adverse reactions in at least two cases. The same document claimed that its distributor had agreed to discontinue selling the product in this country. No word on whether Health Canada managed to entrap him, as he'd so plainly feared they would.

I don't know why it was so hard for me to believe that a wide array of substances ranging from herbs to homeopathics could be used as weapons against such a powerful foe. Indigenous peoples have been using herbs to heal themselves for millennia and the curative properties of homeopathic remedies have been recognized for many centuries. And yet the idea that only a medical doctor could treat a serious illness with a prescription was so ingrained that it wasn't until the medical system let me down so spectacularly that I dipped my toe in other waters.

Those other waters may not have restored my health to what it once was, but they have given me my life back and, as an added bonus, they've made it so that it's been years since I've had to sit across the desk from a doctor who clearly didn't want to be sitting across the desk from me.

Still, like everyone else with advanced Lyme, I keep my eye on the latest medical research, hoping to someday spot the breakthrough that will effectively put an end to entrenched Lyme infections without the need for the prolonged treatment regimes that have become the hallmark of so many Lyme sufferers' lives.

That breakthrough remains unrealized and I suspect that will continue to be the case for several decades. Then again, you never know when a genius moment will arrive and change the course of history.

When I first walked away from the healthcare system in 2007, it was a bit like jumping blind off a cliff. I didn't know whether I was signing my own death warrant or saving my own life. I had no one to advise me, only my own instincts, and they'd been wrong before.

I'd heard of people leaving the healthcare system before — we all have — and watched incredulously as they sought treatment for a serious illness from an alternative practitioner in their hometown, a dubious-sounding medical clinic in an exotic country, or a self-styled healer claiming to have invented a miracle cure in the privacy of his or her own basement laboratory.

I never thought I would be one of those people.

Then I got sick and learned what so many patients before me have learned: universal healthcare is a myth. Healthcare in Canada is reserved for those patients who have the good fortune to suffer from common ailments that don't challenge doctors in any meaningful way.

The rest of us can take a hike.

Suffice to say I grew frustrated with a healthcare system that could not or would not deal with my illness. Doctors were free to insult and/or ignore me as they saw fit. They could refer me to other doctors who would then do the same until there was no place left to refer me. If I still wanted treatment I would have no choice but to loop back to the beginning and start again. Only a fool would expect a different result the second time around.

And then there were public health officials. They seemed to have no qualms about refuting very legitimate concerns over their handling of the Lyme disease issue by questioning whether many of the patients heaping criticism on them even had the disease. Not by their reckoning. And their reckoning ruled the day.

To make matters worse, the doctor whom I encountered through improper channels "voluntarily" retired from practice shortly after I met him, having been bullied by a committee of the College of Physicians and Surgeons of BC to the point where his health began to fail and he could no longer continue to fight for his professional life.

The actions of The College sent a chill through the medical profession in this province.

With no physicians in BC willing to take over this doctor's Lyme patients, it's estimated that close to 200 of them were forced to leave the healthcare system in order to continue treatment. Many sought help from likeminded doctors in the United States or Europe. Others, like me, abandoned conventional medicine and sought help from naturopathic physicians within our own country. Still others turned to home remedies they could administer themselves, as I initially did.

And all because of a medical debate that the patients had no hand in creating.

But we sure paid the price for it.

When I left the healthcare system, I did so knowing that most people wouldn't have made the decision I made. No matter how badly they were treated, no matter how ignorant doctors were, no matter how offensive the statements of public health officials could be, most people simply would never have left the healthcare system to venture out onto a path leading to God knows where.

So what did it take for me to do it? Hubris, to be sure. I mean my own, of course, but if I were to stand on one heel and pivot, I would see hubris in all directions.

Doctors.

Public health officials.

Government regulators.

Licensing boards.

Medical schools.

Many people were responsible for me walking away from the healthcare system and yet the only one who will ever be held accountable for it is me.

And I'm fine with that. You see, the day I left the healthcare system was the day I left the controversy behind. Lyme disease is only controversial within the context of a creaking, shoddy system of medicine that has no capacity to deal with a complex and perplexing illness. Outside of that system, the controversy disappears, except as stories that sometimes crop up in the media and focus on the plight of patients who continue to grapple with a healthcare system that doesn't want them to be a part of it.

It's a sad thing to witness, even when you're witnessing it from afar.

And afar is an excellent place to witness it from.

That's one of the few things I know for certain these days.

PROOF OF LIFE

There are times when it occurs to me that I didn't survive my battle with Lyme disease. I'll be pulling weeds in the garden or placing a pot on the stove and I'll suddenly be struck by the overwhelming sensation that I'm no longer alive. I can even tell you when I died: in the emergency room when my spirit rose above my body and I was able to see myself from a location outside my body for the very first time.

Everything I've experienced since that day has been nothing more than a projection of the life I might've lived if I'd survived. A hallucination spewed by a dying brain. A hallucination that rings so true it's hard to distinguish it from reality. A hallucination that echoes through space and time, buffering my passage from this life to the next one.

That would certainly explain the dream-like quality my life has taken on. Why I have trouble locating my body in three-dimensional space. Why vampires, gargoyles, and magic fairies seem so real, while friends and neighbors seem like apparitions. Why words have no meanings. Why no one has a face. Why I hear and speak in hieroglyphs. Why time moves so slowly. And sometimes goes missing. Why my spirit floats away from my body.

None of this makes sense. It's the stuff of nightmares.

Unless I'm dead. A ghost who cannot accept her own passing. Then all of this makes some sort of sense. I mean, ghosts don't know they're dead, right? They're baffled by the separation between themselves and everything and everyone that was once so accessible to them. An invisible chasm that can't be crossed. That's how it works in the movies, anyways. Someone — a psychic or a priest — needs to get these tormented souls to understand what's happened to them before the balance of the universe is upset, at least as it applies to humankind.

I can't help wondering if the strangeness will be stripped away when I finally accept my fate. If I'll remember my life in a more logical way. Or remember it at all. Remembering isn't exactly my strong suit these days.

For now I'm clinging to this hallucinated life because I don't know what else to cling to and because not clinging to it would mean turning away from what's left of my existence to face what comes next.

But I'm not ready for what comes next. I'm not even ready for what's already here. I don't know why I feel this way. There must be inflammation in a part of my brain responsible for the sensation of being alive, or an imbalance in neurochemicals, or maybe a lack of cerebral blood flow to the reality center of my brain, or maybe even something as mundane as a panic attack. That makes some sort of sense. That doesn't mean it's correct, just rational.

What I wrote about Lyme disease sufferers being misdiagnosed with MS makes no sense if you can simply run a test that will tell you if someone has been infected with Bb, thus ruling out MS as a possible cause for their symptoms. Tests for Lyme disease exist, yes indeed, but instead of clarifying the situation, they have a nasty habit of muddying it.

In Canada, Lyme disease testing is a two-tiered process that begins with an inexpensive, computerized screening test known as an enzyme-linked immunosorbent assay (ELISA). If this test comes up positive or equivocal, a second (more accurate) test called a Western blot is performed in an attempt to confirm the results of the first test. A highly trained technician is needed to interpret the results of this second test, which makes it both more expensive and more labor intensive than the computerized screening test.

The two-tiered testing process was put in place because, in addition to being more expensive to conduct, the Western blot has a reputation for erring on the positive side, so by running the ELISA screening test first, only those samples which are suspicious for Bb make it through to the second phase of testing, reducing the chances that a false positive will be recorded, something that could result in a patient being misdiagnosed with Lyme and unnecessarily treated for a disease they never had.

In theory, this system of testing is accurate 95 percent of the time.

In practice, there are well-documented problems with specificity (a positive result when antibodies to the bacterium are present), sensitivity (a negative result when they aren't), and reproducibility (the same result each time the test is run on a single sample).

Part of the problem has to do with the criteria used to interpret these tests. In Canada, those criteria are set by the Canadian Public Health Laboratory Network (CPHLN) and use the so-called Dearborn criteria as their foundation. These criteria were set, not surprisingly, at a conference held in Dearborn, Michigan in 1994, which sought to standardize the interpretation of Lyme test results so that regardless of which lab does the testing, there would be consistency in what constitutes a positive result.

These criteria have been mired in controversy ever since. Why takes a little explaining.

Attempts at culturing the Bb bacterium in a lab, which would be the ideal, have not proven reliable enough to be used for laboratory diagnosis. Instead we have to settle for the ELISA and Western blot tests, both of which are indirect tests, meaning they don't check for the presence of the Bb bacterium itself, but rather for the antibodies produced by the immune system in response to the bacterium. These antibodies are unique for each organism your body defends itself against, whether it's the flu, the measles, or our dear friend Lyme.

So let's look at those antibodies. The immune system produces two kinds: Immunoglobulin M (IgM) and Immunoglobulin G (IgG). As soon as someone is exposed to Bb (or any other bacteria or virus, for that matter) IgM antibodies are produced. They are a temporary response to an acute attack and two to three weeks after they're produced, they're gone. IgG antibodies, on the other hand, are produced later and stay with you for the rest of your life. It's these IgG antibodies that give you immunity to diseases such as chicken pox or the measles so that you either don't fall ill when you're subsequently exposed to them or you suffer a mild illness.

The Dearborn criteria nailed down which of the dozens of antibodies generated in response to a Bb infection need to be present in order for a test to be considered positive. Ten antibodies were selected and it was decided that five of the ten must be present on the IgG test for it to be positive. Two of three selected antibodies need to be present for a positive result on an IgM test. These banding patterns were (and are) considered highly specific to a Bb infection.

Most of those involved in the Lyme debate agree that the selected antibodies are appropriate. What's in dispute is whether any of the dozens of antibodies not selected as part of the criteria are also diagnostic of a Bb infection, and *only* a Bb infection. Many feel that the selected antibodies are too conservative, leaving out several that only a Bb infection would produce.

Chief among these excluded bands are outer surface protein (Osp)A and OspB. These two antibodies were excluded from the criteria because they were earmarked for the development of vaccines against Lyme and if they'd been included, there would have been no way for the tests to distinguish between someone who'd contracted the disease naturally and someone who'd been vaccinated against it. (It evidently didn't occur to those setting the standards that they could simply ask someone whether or not they'd been vaccinated against the disease prior to running any tests.)

Such a vaccine was indeed developed, but it fizzled and was withdrawn from the market in 2002 after just two years on the market, primarily due to issues surrounding its financial viability, but there were also allegations that it was causing autoimmune-related arthritis and suspiciously Lyme-like symptoms in some of its recipients.

Despite the withdrawal, OspA and OspB continue to be excluded from the diagnostic criteria. So we end up with a strange circumstance. OspA and OspB were excluded from those criteria because if they weren't, patients who had received the vaccine would test positive for an active Lyme infection they likely didn't have. But if a patient does have an active Lyme infection and is reactive on either the OspA or OspB band or both, they won't be considered as having the disease, since neither of these two bands will be taken into account when the test results are being interpreted.

It's enough to make your head spin.

I wake up and I'm relieved to find myself lying in bed and not on the floor. I'm dazed and nauseous and have the sort of skull-cracking headache normally associated with a hangover. I try to work out what led to this moment and, considering I haven't had a drop of alcohol in more than a year, I'm guessing it wasn't the wild whiskey-fest that my head is now claiming.

A clue is written on the inside of my eyelids.

That clue looks something like the engineering schematics for an alien spacecraft. These schematics have been drawn in phosphorescent light and as I lie in bed — eyes closed, brain screaming — I study the complicated geometric patterns glowing against my eyelids. Straight arrows. Jagged lines. Tilted triangles. Tipsy rectangles.

These brilliant, basic shapes are jumbled together as if someone upended the box containing them and, like a belligerent child, left them lying in tangles on the inside of my eyelids.

That's the least of it.

My spinal fluid is effervescing. At first it's just in my neck, but then the fizzing starts creeping down my spine. When it hits my tailbone, it violently reverses course and thousands of tiny bubbles shoot furiously upwards, colliding with the base of my skull.

Pain shoots towards my left ear and the left side of my face is reduced to numb rubber. My jaw locks and the teeth on the left side of my mouth disappear, while the beast in my chest pulls hard on the root of my tongue in a desperate bid to drag it backwards down my throat.

And then there are my fingers. They're tingling in the most unusual way. I raise them in front of my eyes, half-expecting them to shoot stars. Half expecting them to be made of stars.

Why is this happening? Who knows?

I can't seem to concentrate.

The bubbles are forcing their way through the base of my skull. They swirl across the surface of my brain like dozens of tiny hurricanes, spilling nausea and weakness down the left side of my body.

These boiling bubbles leak into my eyes. They stream across a flat, gray panel that breaks free and floats up diagonally out of my visual field only to be replaced by another panel that also breaks free and floats away.

This again. Only not exactly. The air freezes before my eyes.

And there's silence. I don't mean to suggest there's a complete loss of sound. I'm not deaf. It's more like the tense silence you hear when a barn full of chickens suddenly realizes there's a coyote at the gate.

Something's coming.

Let's take a moment to consider how timing affects the accuracy of Lyme tests.

The ELISA screening test has well-documented problems with accuracy when it's performed within four weeks of a tick bite and because of this, negative test results must be confirmed with a follow-up ELISA test approximately one month after the first. If that second ELISA throws a positive result, then the more accurate Western blot will be performed to confirm it.

Got that?

This, of course, means that if you're bitten by an infected tick and develop a nasty looking rash — that rash public health officials do so love to go on about — and are given a Lyme test while that rash is still fresh, that test stands an excellent chance of coming back negative even though you're in all likelihood infected with Lyme disease. That's because the ELISA is accurate less than 50 percent of the time during those critical first four weeks after infection when, ironically, treatment stands the best chance of being effective.

This one fact alone makes it critical that doctors be able to diagnose Lyme clinically. By the time the ELISA test stands a good chance of being accurate, the window for successful treatment has already passed.

So then, once those first four weeks pass, the ELISA screening test magically becomes more accurate, right? Well, not exactly. The problems with the screening test don't disappear after those initial four weeks are up; I don't mean to suggest that. It's estimated that the screening test continues to miss approximately 50 percent of cases — there is, of course, some dispute over the exact percentage — when it's conducted more than a month after initial infection, all thanks to known sensitivity issues that make the screening test more of a crapshoot than a definitive diagnostic tool.

The obvious question is, why? Well, for one, it's been discovered that roughly 20 percent of people infected with Bb never develop antibodies to the infection and many of those who do, produce so few that both the ELISA and Western blot tests are rendered ineffective. Remember, these tests check for antibodies to Bb, not for the actual bacteria, so if your body doesn't try to defend itself against the invading bacteria — if it doesn't recognize our diabolical friend as being an invader but rather thinks it's whatever kind of body cell it's trying so hard to disguise itself as — then no antibodies will be produced and there's nothing for the test to find.

This alone would certainly help to explain why such a large percentage of cases are missed.

But it isn't alone.

Another complication — because with Lyme there must always be another complication — is that any patient who has been treated with antibiotics prior to an ELISA test being conducted stands a good chance of receiving a negative test result as a consequence of that treatment even though they may not truly be free of infection. The treatment may have simply reduced an already low antibody count, leading to a negative test result that could very well be contradicted by a second test done at a later date, if such a test is ever conducted.

Don't hold your breath on that one. It's hard enough to get a doctor to order the first round of testing.

And all of this is problematic. An immune system that doesn't create antibodies at all or in large enough quantities that they can be measured on the screening test will cause that test to report that there are no antibodies present in the sample and it will be correct. It's just unfortunate that the absence of antibodies does not always equate to an absence of Bb.

I open my eyes and immediately wish I hadn't. Everything I see—ceiling, air, sunlight—is hewn from undulating iridescent light. As I watch the world languidly twist and warp, I try to work out if this is the same day that the phosphorescent schematics appeared on the inside of my eyelids or if a week, a month, or even a year has passed in the interim. I can't tell if a second has passed or a decade, but I can tell that the wall in front of me is folding in on itself. So is the air, my body, even my thoughts.

I hold my hand out in front of my face and watch as it melts into the air surrounding it.

And I think this: What's stopping my hand from melting into the wall?

More than melting into it. What's stopping my hand from passing through the wall and bringing the rest of my body with it? This thought requires investigation. I throw back the sheets, raise my arms out in front of me like a B-movie zombie, then aim for the wall, curious to see if I can melt into it, through it, past it. I give it a try.

I'm left with the vague feeling I may have succeeded. I can't quite remember. I wish I could.

Many observers have noted that the awesome genetic diversity of Bb may be yet another wild card affecting test accuracy for Lyme disease.

There are more than 100 known strains of Bb in North America (300 worldwide) and researchers are certain that more are waiting to be discovered. So it's not surprising to learn that studies have been undertaken looking at whether the accuracy of Lyme disease testing in Canada is being affected by the way in which Bb spread across the continent.

Because assumptions were made. And it turns out those assumptions were wrong. Specifically, it's long been assumed that Bb was spreading westward from endemic regions in the northeastern United States. However, recent findings are throwing that assumption into question. Big time.

Evidence now suggests that instead of spreading from east to west, Bb is spreading from south to north, meaning that the strains of the bacterium found in British Columbia are more likely to be related to those found in California, Oregon or Washington State than those found in the New England states or even the Midwest.

There's also evidence to suggest that Bb has been making its home in Canada for long enough now that indigenous populations are starting to evolve independently from populations found outside of Canada, something that could mean there are strains present in this country that are unique in the world.

Yet we don't produce our own Lyme test kits in this country. This means that Lyme tests conducted in Canada haven't been optimized for the strains of Bb present in this country. And when labs in Canada use Lyme tests kits that were developed in the United States or Europe, those kits could conceivably be causing problems since they're optimized for foreign strains of the bacterium and could therefore generate negative results for someone infected with a Bb strain far removed from the ones found in the Lyme hot spots of northeastern United States or Europe.

That begs the following question: Of the 100 or so strains of Bb known to exist in North America, which strain (or strains) dominate in the region of Canada where you live? Throw a dart and maybe you'll get an answer. Otherwise you'll have to wait until more research is conducted.

Initial studies suggest that novel strains may indeed be at play in Canada and a whole lot more work needs to be done in this area before a clear picture develops of just how diverse the genetic picture is in this country.

So stay tuned. Interesting findings are surely on the horizon.

There's another question that needs to be asked here, an important one: What if a patient's case of Lyme disease is caused by a borrelia species other than Bb? *Borrelia bavariensis*, say, or possibly *Borrelia spielmanii?*

Traditionally, Lyme testing in Canada recognized Bb sensu stricto as the causative agent of Lyme, and only recently has that been shifted to include Bb sensu lato. But again, the fact remains there may be borrelia species present in Canada that are novel to this country, something that researchers are trying to confirm. Does that make a difference? Maybe, maybe not.

Cross-reactivity is a known problem with Lyme testing. Cross-reactivity happens because although the antibodies we produce are unique for each organism that attacks us, the ELISA test has difficulty distinguishing between those antibodies directed against Bb and those directed against organisms closely related to Bb due to the antigens these organisms share in common. Cross-reactivity has the potential to make it so that novel strains of Bb and borrelia species other than Bb can trigger positive results on Lyme tests targeting specific strains of Bb.

Of course, the opposite can also happen and someone infected with a species of borrelia other than Bb can end up with all the symptoms of Lyme and yet come up negative on the antibody tests because cross-reactivity failed to rear its ugly head.

And cross-reactivity can cause other challenges for test accuracy. If you're infected with syphilis or relapsing tick fever and are tested for Lyme, a false positive can be triggered on the Lyme screening test. A false positive can also be triggered if you're infected with hepatitis A, herpes simplex, mononucleosis or HIV, are suffering from rheumatoid arthritis or lupus, or, sometimes, if you simply have elevated inflammatory proteins. The more accurate Western blot test would then help determine whether the positive result is a true positive.

Not that the Western blot is bulletproof, either. I mean, there's a reason why the manufacturers of the Lyme test kits (ELISA and Western blot) include disclaimers instructing technicians that negative tests cannot be used to definitively rule out the Lyme, and positive tests should not be taken as clear proof that Lyme is present. These tests are fallible and that's problematic for anyone hoping that testing will yield a definitive answer for whether someone does or does not have a Lyme infection. By anyone, I mean doctors.

Which leads me to wonder why, if the manufacturers of the test kits aren't confident that their kits will yield firm results, should anyone else be?

I've spent much of the last year lying on the floor of my loft, staring up at the vaulted ceiling that the previous owner painted an inexplicable shade of blue. Powder blue, to be exact. Now there's a color one doesn't expect to see splashed across manly wooden beams.

I'm once again lying on that floor. I have an EpiPen in one hand, while the other is resting on an artery in my neck. My heart is ticking down like a time bomb.

It's not the desperately slow heart rate that concerns me. What concerns me is that when my heart rate drops below sixty beats per minute it starts to behave erratically. From fifty beats per minute, it plummets to thirty beats, slingshots back up to a normal rate, then stops beating altogether before bouncing up to thirty beats again.

When my heart stops beating altogether there's a sensation of floating, an ethereal calm, and I lie here wondering how many missed beats I should wait before jamming epinephrine into my thigh. It'll certainly make my heart beat faster.

I'm just not entirely sure that's a good thing. I mean, in the movies they stab a needle full of adrenaline straight into the heart muscle to reverse heart failure, so there's reason to believe it might work. But shooting epinephrine into the thigh isn't quite the same as shooting adrenaline into the heart.

It could set up a dangerous arrhythmia. Not that I don't already have one.

Still, I have to do something and I just can't face a trip to the emergency room. So I grip the EpiPen in my hand and try not to think about how this will read on the death certificate. "Death by misadventure" would be my preference, but corpses don't generally get a vote in these sorts of things.

I'm not done with the tests yet.

There's also a question of reproducibility surrounding both the ELISA and Western blot tests.

Several studies have shown that when identical samples are sent to different labs there is a high degree of variability in the results that are returned. Part of this variability is blamed on the criteria used to interpret the tests, criteria that were developed in research labs, not diagnostic ones. Critics have long questioned the technical ability of diagnostic labs to produce accurate results using commercial kits.

The variability is also blamed on the kits being used. More than 70 diagnostic test kits have been approved by the U.S. Food and Drug Administration (FDA) for the detection of Bb antibodies and these kits have been shown to lack standardization, causing their ability to detect antibodies to vary greatly, not just between kits from different manufacturers, mind you, but also between batches of kits from the same manufacturer. That would certainly explain a few things.

Yet technical deficits don't get the whole blame.

One of the many complaints about Lyme testing is that it hasn't changed significantly in more than a decade, a time period during which a host of new developments have occurred in other areas of Lyme research, developments that together are leading to a better understanding of the Lyme organism(s). Yet advances in testing are failing to keep pace, something that seems foolhardy when you consider that Lyme disease infections worldwide are increasing at a breathtaking rate.

There are few positive signs in this area, but one of the positive signs would have to be Health Canada's recent approval of the C6 peptide ELISA test in Canada. This test is considered to be more accurate than the standard ELISA that has dominated Canadian testing for many years. It's still an antibody test and therefore subject to the same issues affecting other antibody tests for Lyme — something that makes it a small step forward indeed — but a small step forward is still a step in the right direction. Ideally these antibody tests will one day be abandoned for a better technology.

We just need to wait until someone develops that technology.

This brings us to an even bigger problem facing Lyme testing in Canada.

A significant drawback to the two-tiered testing system used in this country is the requirement that the ELISA be positive or equivocal before a Western blot can be performed. This means that if the ELISA comes up negative, no Western blot is ever performed to verify the result, taking away an important fail-safe.

This leaves a lot of patients in the lurch. Think about it. Anyone whose body never produced antibodies to the infection or produced only a few, who is treated with antibiotics prior to testing, who is tested too early, who is in an advanced state when tested, who currently has a distinctive EM rash, or who just plain has bad luck runs the risk of being told that they don't have Lyme disease based solely on the results of an unconfirmed negative screening test.

One thing most of the participants involved in the Lyme disease debate can agree on is that Lyme should be diagnosed based on clinical symptoms and exposure to infected ticks, not test results. There are just too many problems with existing testing to rely on it to definitively establish whether a patient does or does not have the disease. Unfortunately, most doctors aren't involved in the Lyme debate and remain largely unaware of the significant problems with testing, assuming instead that diagnostic tests wouldn't be in use if they're known to have such glaring deficits.

So then, an important question needs to be asked: How does a doctor go about clinically diagnosing Lyme disease when there is no consensus among experts on just what its symptoms might be with the exception of an EM rash that as few as 20 percent of sufferers ever see?

A crystal ball might make things easier. Or divine intervention.

A process of elimination is certainly required to rule out other causes, but when a patient's symptoms mimic a disease that's far more common than Lyme — lupus, for instance — then that patient stands an excellent chance of being diagnosed with the more common illness without Lyme being given a second thought.

To make things more interesting, existing guidelines strongly suggest that a doctor only consider Lyme disease if a patient lives in, or has visited, an area considered endemic for Lyme disease. And yet, as I pointed out in chapter 16, 85 percent of Ontario residents who contracted Lyme within that province between 2002 and 2006 had never visited an endemic region.

Consider as well that ticks known to carry Bb have been found in northern Alberta and the Yukon, neither of which has ever been listed as endemic for the bacterium, making existing guidelines out of step with the realities of Lyme disease in this country. If you can contract Lyme in the Yukon — and the presence of the ticks that carry Bb makes that possible — then all of Canada is in play, regardless of whether breeding tick populations have been found in specific regions or not. Visiting ticks are just as capable of spreading infection as resident ones.

So what happens if someone feels that the results they received on the ELISA test for Lyme disease may have been falsely negative due to one or more of the myriad problems affecting the accuracy of these tests? With no recourse in Canada other than to have the same problematic tests performed again and again, many turn to commercial labs in the United States that specialize in testing for tick-borne illnesses.

These labs offer medical refugees a few things not available to them in Canada.

First off, they give them access to the more accurate Western blot test that can only be accessed in Canada when a positive or equivocal test result is recorded on the ELISA screening test. In having the tests redone in the USA, patients gain the opportunity to have a Western blot test confirm or contradict the results of the ELISA screening test.

These labs also give patients access to something that's more intriguing: They use a standard of interpretation that's more liberal than the controversial Dearborn criteria adhered to by labs in Canada. Specifically, several of these labs include the two antibodies — OspA and OspB — that were set aside for the development of vaccines. Some also include a series of antibodies that research has shown to be implicated in the chronic and recurrent forms of Lyme, antibodies that were also excluded from the Dearborn criteria in spite of the concerns expressed by leading researchers that their exclusion would give negative results to many people who really do have the disease.

Lyme disease tests performed by specialized labs in the US throw the net wider, to be sure, and labs that conform to the more conservative Dearborn criteria (including government-operated labs in Canada) complain that they throw the net too wide, returning positive results to patients who wouldn't receive them under the standardized criteria. This may be true, but then the tests for Lyme disease have never been conclusive and these labs do have a legitimate rationale for their divergence from the Dearborn criteria. And in performing a Western blot regardless of the ELISA result, they provide an important fail-safe against false negative results that's currently lacking in Canada.

Since Lyme tests are supposed to be nothing more than a single piece of information — like clinical symptoms or exposure risk — to be taken into consideration when arriving at a diagnosis, then the differences in the interpretation criteria shouldn't make all that much difference. The problem is that these tests are being seen by doctors as much more than that. They're being seen as definitive diagnostic tools, clearly answering the question whether or not a patient has Lyme, and that's a claim that not even the manufacturers of these tests are willing to assert.

Neither should anyone else.

Now why would I care about any of this? My own ELISA and Western blot tests — both of which were performed in 2007 by a government laboratory using the more stringent Dearborn criteria — came back positive. I also live in an area known to be endemic for Lyme disease and had traveled to other Lyme-endemic areas prior to being diagnosed with Lyme. And — show-off that I can sometimes be — I had a collection of symptoms that caused the illness to make it onto the radar of at least one of the doctors tasked with trying to figure out what was wrong with me.

In short, I had what few other Lyme sufferers in Canada ever have: a rock-solid case of Lyme disease that both doctors and public health officials agree on. Whatever the deficits in Lyme testing may be, those tests appeared to work just fine for me. So then why am I taking the time to highlight the problems with Lyme testing in such detail when I could've just noted them in passing and moved on to something significantly less geeky?

Because in addition to being diagnosed with Lyme disease, I was diagnosed with a second tick-borne infection: relapsing tick fever. But then you already knew that, didn't you? I told you that in the first part of this book and although I haven't mentioned it since, I never did say that that diagnosis had been rescinded.

What happened with relapsing tick fever is far more interesting than that.

And, if you're patient, I'll tell you why.

The textile bleaching agent is having an effect.

The question, of course, is whether the effect it's having is the result of killing toxin-spewing bacteria or whether it's slowly poisoning the life right out of me. I fear it could be the latter, but I don't alter course because, if nothing else, what's happening now is familiar.

Third-week-of-antibiotics familiar. Yes, it feels like the same thing that happened when the antibiotics finally kicked in, only more pronounced.

Not that that necessarily means anything. Maybe dying has a familiar feeling to it. Maybe it feels the same regardless of the cause.

How would I know? And would it really matter?

The goal of this whole exercise is to bring the suffering to an end and when you think about it, killing bacteria or killing me will both accomplish the desired result so, one way or another, I'm making great strides towards achieving my goal.

I can't remember the last time that was true.

A TICK IN THE OINTMENT

I'm sitting on the edge of the bed, trying to determine whether or not my feet are touching the floor. That's the problem with perpetually numb feet. I actually need to see the floor, then see where my feet are in relation to it, in order to determine whether or not the two are connecting.

There's no other way to tell.

Anyway, the floor and my feet aren't connecting and while I'm looking down I notice that a blue-black bruise has engulfed my baby toe and the outer third of my foot. I turn my foot sole-side up and discover that the entire ball of my foot is the same breathtaking shade of blue. Cadaver blue. Whatever else a blue foot is, it's psychologically damaging.

Where the sole isn't blue, it's covered with pale splotches that look like albino bruises. These splotches are the size of dimes except for where they gang together on my heel in an unruly flock. My first thought is that I must've done something to injure my foot. A ghost of a memory is telling me that I may have slammed my foot into a table leg during a recent shaking fit.

It's hard to say for sure. Remembering what happens during these fits is like remembering the details of a dream I had while lying drunk at the bottom of a swimming pool, so I try instead to determine when I think my foot may or may not have whomped the table leg.

Yesterday?

Maybe.

Or last week?

This is futile.

If I could feel my foot, I might be able to narrow things down a bit. Pain can be a valuable clue.

But there is no pain. There's no feeling at all.

And I have my doubts about the whole injury theory. Bruised body parts usually look offended by what's been done to them, especially when the insult spans so much territory. But my foot doesn't look particularly offended. It looks as though someone inserted a straw into my big toe and sucked all the air out of it and I find this fascinating.

I poke at both kinds of bruises — cadaver and albino — and discover that it's a bit like poking at the skin of a defrosted turkey. My flesh has been replaced by a lifeless gel that I can pinch and prod and reposition like modeling compound.

In a way, I'm relieved. I'd almost thought I was going to make it through an entire day without my body doing something gross or horrifying, but no, the status quo has once again been preserved. Thank God for that. It may not be desirable, but at least it's predictable and the only comfort I can find these days is in the predictability of the chaos.

I should probably do something about the blue foot. I decide not to walk to the bathroom out of fear that the weight of my body might crush something inside my foot that can't later be uncrushed.

So I crawl. It's nothing the rafters haven't witnessed before and eventually I reach the bathroom, where I fill the sink with warm water, then perch on the counter with my shoulders against the towel rod, bracing as I lower my foot into the water.

I don't know what I'm bracing for. Whatever it is, it doesn't arrive. The blue slowly melts away and is replaced by a bright, splashy red that covers my foot and ankle. Fruit-punch red. I feel like the subject of an Impressionist painting.

I wonder if I should try walking on my fruit-punch foot. I don't want to risk permanent damage, but I also don't want to perch on the counter for the rest of my life.

I wish this disease came with a rulebook. A user's manual. Everything would be so much easier if I could just turn to the page that says, "When your feet turn blue, dunk them in warm water, but absolutely do not place any weight on them. When your feet turn fruit-punch red, walk on them sparingly. Whenever your feet can be seen but not felt, watch out for sudden face-punchings by solid wood floors." Now that would be some helpful advice.

Let's return to the subject of relapsing tick fever, an illness that's rarely mentioned in the same breath as Lyme disease and yet ranks as the one tick-borne illness that I've grown to know as well as I know Lyme.

Relapsing tick fever is occasionally mistaken for other illnesses. Those illnesses include Rocky Mountain spotted fever, malaria, typhoid fever, brucellosis, dengue fever, bacterial meningitis, and Colorado tick fever.

It can also be mistaken for Lyme disease.

These mistakes are made by doctors with little or no experience in dealing with relapsing tick fever, which just happens to be most doctors. Experts, on the other hand, point out that the fevers it manifests are unlike those of any other disease.

But relapsing tick fever is extremely rare, far rarer than Lyme. Just 450 cases were recorded in the United States over a period of 14 years ending in 2006 and those figures have remained relatively stable for more than 50 years. The number of cases in Canada is significantly lower than that, roughly two to four cases per year, largely because the only place in Canada where the illness is known to occur is in the Rocky Mountain region of southeastern and south-central British Columbia where relapsing tick fever has traditionally been more prevalent than Lyme disease.

So then I guess it's not all that surprising to discover that almost one-third of patients suffering from relapsing tick fever in the United States and Canada experience at least two fever episodes before doctors clue into the cause of their illness, largely because they hadn't considered it as a possibility up to that point.

Like relapsing tick fever, Lyme disease is known to cause fevers.

Unlike relapsing tick fever, Lyme fevers are usually persistent and low-grade. Sometimes they spike higher, but Lyme fevers rarely go above 39C and they certainly don't recur and remit in the dramatic way relapsing tick fevers do.

You can set your watch by relapsing tick fevers.

You can bookmark important dates by them.

Here's an important date to bookmark: 1933. That's the year the first outbreak of relapsing tick fever was reported in British Columbia. The infections all occurred between 1930 and 1932 in the Lower Arrow Lake region of the West Kootenays.

I could hit that region with a rock from here.

All told, six cases were eventually identified in that initial outbreak. Then, in 1937, a couple of loggers turned up with the disease in the Okanagan Valley community of Vernon and, if you fast-forward all the way to 1984, you'll discover that two more cases were identified in that same locale.

In recent decades, a handful of cases each year have become the norm.

A type of borrelia bacteria, *Borrelia hermsii* (Bh, for short) was assumed to be the causative agent in all of those early outbreaks, but it was only in the three cases that later occurred in the south Okanagan in the mid-1990s that the exact species of borrelia was confirmed by laboratory analysis.

Bh wasn't the only option.

Relapsing tick fever is caused by more than a dozen closely related bacteria that are contracted from the bite of an infected tick. These bacteria all belong to the borrelia genus, a genus that's broken down into two groups causing illness in humans: those associated with relapsing tick fever and those associated with Lyme disease. (There are other types of borrelia that aren't known to cause illness in humans.)

The species of borrelia that cause relapsing tick fever have traditionally been named for the ticks they infest, which have long been presumed to be their natural vectors. *Borrelia hermsii*, for instance, is the species that infests *Ornithodorus hermsi* ticks while *Borrelia parkeri* infests *Ornithodorus parkeri* ticks.

It's all rather orderly.

All rather scientific.

So then it's not surprising that there's a mountain of research that says relapsing tick fever is carried by soft-bodied, night-feeding, argasid (Ornithodoros) ticks. And yet when those original cases of relapsing tick fever were described in the 1930s, no Ornithodoros ticks had ever been found in Canada. As a result, Dermacentor ticks were initially blamed for the outbreak.

It would be almost two decades before *Ornithodorus hermsi* specimens were finally collected from a bird nest in Summerland, BC. It was a landmark discovery because the "natural" vector for relapsing tick fever had finally been found in BC. Who cares if it was many years after the fact? Apparently someone did, because a 1986 report pointed out that although, yes indeed, *O. hermsi* ticks had been collected in Canada, not one of those ticks had ever been proven to be infected with Bh, something that makes the assertion that cases of relapsing tick fever in British Columbia are caused exclusively by Bh bacteria vectored into humans by Ornithodoros ticks little more than an assumption.

A logical assumption, true enough.

But it doesn't rule out the possibility that those original cases of relapsing tick fever really could have been caused by the bites of Dermacentor ticks, as initially reported, carrying a species of relapsing fever borrelia — possibly Bh, possibly something else — and it doesn't rule out the possibility that some of the cases of relapsing tick fever being diagnosed today are also being caused by species of borrelia other than Bh.

Canadian research in this area is largely absent.

Relapsing tick fever is named for its dominant symptom: a dramatic recurring fever that's unique in the world of illness. It arrives without warning and can last anywhere from one to three days, during which time it easily blasts past 40C, then spikes and recedes multiple times.

Then it goes into remission. The fever disappears. The patient starts to feel better. She starts to feel almost human. Almost.

Then one day — maybe several days, maybe several weeks later — the fever makes a dramatic return and the cycle repeats. Untreated, these fever periods can return a dozen times, and they always end in a crisis that typically involves the abrupt arrival of shaking chills, extreme high fevers, a rapid pulse, high blood pressure and excessive sweating followed by plummeting body temperatures and blood pressure.

And that's not all.

Relapsing tick fever can cause all sorts of problems in addition to the fever, such as inflammation of the nerve roots, heart, brain and spinal cord (and the coverings of both). Symptoms can include total paralysis of an arm, a leg or one side of the body, weakness or impairment of the upper or lower extremities, an unsteady gait, absent reflexes, headaches, backaches, a stiff neck, vertigo, tinnitus, hearing loss or deafness, wide-ranging vision problems, facial palsy, tremors, muscle and joint pain, abdominal pain, language impairment, persistent and/or extreme fatigue, anorexia, nausea, enlarged spleen, vomiting, coughing, delirium, hallucinations, mania, seizures, jaundice, respiratory problems, sensitivity to light, confusion, jaundice, and non-specific rashes. Relapsing tick fever can even cause hemorrhaging.

It sounds like a terrible disease. It also sounds like a familiar one.

Some of the symptoms listed above are common, others are rare, but all are possible. Which ones a patient develops is determined largely by his or her body's own unique inflammatory response and by which species of borrelia he or she comes into contact with, which can vary significantly in the severity of illness they induce, and the number of clinical relapses.

These distinctive relapsing fevers occur because the borrelia species that cause relapsing tick fever — and there are quite a few of them worldwide — behave very much like the ones that cause Lyme disease when they find themselves under attack.

Why wouldn't they?

The bacteria that cause relapsing tick fever and those that cause Lyme disease are, after all, closely related members of the same family. So when the immune system launches an attack against relapsing tick fever bacteria, the majority are killed. Any that aren't alter their outer surface proteins — they don diabolical disguises — so that they no longer appear to be the invading organisms they are.

The immune system responds by breaking off the attack, believing the enemy to have been defeated. The fever recedes and so do the symptoms that came with it. The patient starts to feel better. She starts to feel almost human. Almost.

Then the immune system realizes it's been duped. It launches a renewed attack, this time targeting the altered bacteria, which have started to increase in numbers, causing the fever to return, along with any and all of the symptoms that came with it the first time around. The bacteria respond to the attack by once again altering their surface proteins — donning different diabolical disguises — and once again the immune system is convinced it's been victorious.

And once again it's wrong.

Untreated, these fever episodes can recur a dozen times before they finally cease. They stop because one of several things happens: the immune system has been successful in defeating the bacteria; antibiotics have been introduced and assist the immune system in annihilating the bacteria; the immune system no longer recognizes the altered bacteria as a threat; the patient dies.

That last one doesn't happen very often. Although worldwide the mortality rate for relapsing fevers can be anywhere from two to 40 percent, depending on the species of borrelia involved and the age of the patient, the tick-borne varieties in North America tend to boast a more conservative death rate in the zero to eight percent range. And if you're bitten by an infected tick in the Kootenay region of British Columbia, it's assumed you'll contract *Borrelia hermsii*, which comes in at the low end of the mortality scale. Not surprisingly, that's the species that was assumed to have infected me.

However, although it was suspected as the agent of relapsing tick fever cases in British Columbia all the way back to the 1930s, Bh was not actually confirmed as the cause in any case until three patients involved in an outbreak in the South Okanagan between 1995 and 1996 were shown to be infected with that particular borrelia species. The exact cause of relapsing tick fever in all previous cases remains unknown.

Possibly *Borrelia parkeri* was the infecting agent in some of those cases. Possibly it was something else. Nobody really knows. That's pretty tenuous stuff to be basing an assumption on, if you ask me.

Long-held assumptions in the area of borrelia infections in Canada are in the process of being re-evaluated pretty much across the board, so it wouldn't surprise me if some future study implicates a species of borrelia other than Bh in some of the cases of relapsing tick fever in British Columbia.

It's practically guaranteed.

No body part should ever be blue unless it's intentionally dyed that color. I'd like to declare my position on that subject right now on the off chance that my body is still even remotely interested in what I think.

Doubtful. It's too busy rebelling to consider my declarations as anything other than a nuisance.

The shocking shade of blue isn't limited to my feet; that's just where the effect is the most dramatic. My fingers and palms also trend towards cadaver hues, although they like to turn more of a gunmetal-gray than a true deathly blue. On bad days, that gray extends up my left arm, so that when I place my two arms side-by-side they appear to belong to two different people: one living, the other dead.

Maybe I'm morphing into a zombie.

If I were a twelve-year-old boy that would probably strike me as a pretty cool thing to do. But I'm not a twelve-year-old boy — not by a long shot — so mostly I just find it alarming.

It's the hands that bother me the most because, short of wearing mittens all day long, there's no way I can escape the sight of them. I can hide my feet in socks and shroud my arm in a sleeve, but my hands? They get submerged in water for as long as it takes them to fade to a somewhat human shade and there they briefly plateau before returning to their customary blue.

Then it's back to the sink.

They must think I'm trying to drown them.

Maybe I am.

At least I'm doing something constructive to combat the hand problem.

That's not true of my arm.

I can find nothing that will turn it a normal color once it goes gray and I have serious concerns that one day soon it will start to rot from the lack of blood flow. I mean, I try not to think about that.

I try to think positive thoughts. But seriously, you should see the color this thing turns. It looks like something you'd pull from a dumpster behind a hospital in some third world country.

It looks inhuman.

It looks unholy.

So I hide it in a sleeve and tell myself that there isn't a single problem in this world that can be solved by hyperventilating.

When I was diagnosed with both Lyme disease and relapsing tick fever, I found that doctors of all stripes were either unwilling or unable to give me any satisfactory information about either disease. Other than telling me the name of the illnesses and that symptoms could get worse — possibly even life-threatening — once treatment began, I was told nothing.

In fact, with the exception of that one frightfully well-informed doctor I came in contact with through improper channels, not one doctor seemed to know enough about either disease to have anything intelligent to say about them. And the frightfully well-informed doctor only wanted to discuss Lyme disease, dismissing relapsing tick fever as a nuisance or possibly a misdiagnosis.

So I had little choice but to do my own research if I wanted to discover how these two diseases behave when they manifest in a single host. After all, it's well known that Lyme behaves in one way when it arrives on its own and quite another when it brings along a co-infection. The two (or more) infections can join forces. They can gang together in biofilm communities. They can swap genetic information back and forth, creating a microbial behemoth. The result is a conglomerated illness that can be so much more than the sum of its parts. When Lyme and babesia get together, as I mentioned earlier, they create a third illness that tends to be both more severe and more enduring than the individual infections that gave rise to it.

So I hit the books.

Then I hit a wall. Books and articles on Lyme disease tend to have a lot to say about co-infections. They list the types of symptoms that can arise from co-infections with babesia, bartonella, anaplasma, rickettsia, and/or various other organisms, often in great detail. But they don't mention relapsing tick fever.

And resources on relapsing tick fever rarely mention Lyme disease. I could find nothing to connect the two illnesses and you've probably already twigged to why: Lyme disease and relapsing tick fever, though related bacterially, are unrelated entomologically. Or, to put it simply, they infect two different types of ticks. Conventional wisdom says that the only way I could have contracted both illnesses was to have been bitten by two ticks of two different species, each carrying a rare tick-borne illness, and the chances of that being the case are infinitesimal.

The law of averages says don't bet on it. There's no realistic chance of overlap between the two diseases.

So then how did I get diagnosed with both? The simplest answer is that the doctor who handed down the diagnosis didn't realize there was anything extraordinary about it and neither did the subsequent doctors who nodded their heads meaningfully and didn't contradict their colleague. Test results, clinical symptoms, risk exposure — all evidence seemed to support the dual diagnosis.

Well, sort of.

When I was tested for the main bacterium that causes Lyme — *Borrelia burgdorferi* — both the ELISA screening test and the Western blot test came back positive. When I was tested for *Borrelia hermsii* — the bacterium known to cause relapsing tick fever in British Columbia — the screening test (which is known as an IFA test, and considered to be more accurate than an ELISA test) came back positive, but the Western blot came back negative. No spirochetes were seen in either case and relapsing tick fever is often conclusively diagnosed by the presence of spirochetes in blood smears. (Spirochetes are rarely seen in Lyme disease.)

If we ignore clinical symptoms and risk exposure and look only at the test results, they appear to show exposure only to Bb. The positive result for Bh on the screening test (which the Western blot failed to confirm) suggests that the screening test for antibodies to relapsing tick fever was cross-reactive: The presence of antibodies to Bb caused false positive results on the Bh screening test, something that's always a possibility on these tests.

The tests appeared to work as they were designed. Lyme disease could be ruled in. Relapsing tick fever could be ruled out. But only if we isolate the test results from all other criteria.

The main problem with doing that is the clinical symptoms said something quite different. That distinctive fever I'd been suffering from was extremely atypical for Lyme disease. In fact, it was extremely atypical for most illnesses on this planet known to cause fevers.

Doctors couldn't help but comment on it. Neither could public health officials.

Malaria had been ruled out. So had typhoid. One by one, every illness that could cause a remitting/recurring fever fell by the wayside until just one was left standing: The second illness had to be relapsing tick fever. It fit clinically. It fit geographically. It (kind of) fit serologically.

And so the diagnosis of Lyme disease and relapsing tick fever stuck like Krazy Glue. It appeared as though I'd managed to do the unexpected, if not quite the impossible: I'd managed to get myself bitten by two ticks of two different species, each carrying a relatively rare tick-borne illness.

Improbable? Absolutely. But as any ten-year-old can tell you, improbable and impossible aren't the same things.

And I do, by some odd quirk of fate, happen to live in the only region in Canada endemic for both Lyme disease and relapsing tick fever, which increases the odds that a dual infection could have occurred. Of course, the reality is that those odds only increase from virtually non-existent to marginally above virtually non-existent.

The thermometer is no longer in danger of sprouting a mushroom cloud.

For the longest time, I took my temperature to monitor just how high the fevers were rocketing in case I needed to take steps to knock them back. (Which I rarely did, so I don't know why I bothered with the thermometer.) But the fevers that once plagued me have vanished and, just for a laugh, busted my internal thermostat on their way out.

My body temperature now chronically hovers at just a hair below 35˚C. Cold radiates from my bones. Sometimes I shake uncontrollably and yet all that shaking fails to produce any heat. It just makes me tired and confused and desperate for something, anything, that will bring just a hint of warmth. So I pile on sweaters and wrap myself in blankets, waiting for a St. Bernard to arrive with a caskful of brandy, which I won't be able to drink, but at least I can look at it.

And I can hug the beast that brought it.

The one possibility that can't be ignored is that my official diagnosis is wrong.

There's an assumption being made — based largely on the presence of a bizarre remitting-recurring fever and my location in the Rocky Mountains — that the Western blot for relapsing tick fever must've thrown a false negative. By the same token, another possibility must be considered: That the test for Lyme disease may have done the opposite and thrown a false positive.

Lyme information rarely mentions relapsing tick fever except to note that the tests for Lyme can throw false positives if relapsing tick fever is present. Resources on relapsing tick fever have a bit more to say on the subject. For instance, one study looked at 182 cases of relapsing tick fever and noted that most patients with relapsing tick fever came up positive on blood tests for Lyme disease and not just on the screening test. The Lyme Western blot, which is considered the more accurate of the two tests, commonly threw false positives when a patient was truly infected with relapsing tick fever. The study's authors concluded that because of this, cases of relapsing tick fever in the northwestern United States and southwestern Canada are no doubt being misdiagnosed as Lyme disease. Many other researchers agree.

It gets even better.

Some of those researchers have suggested that relapsing tick fever is such a rare disease that if a lab that doesn't have a test kit on hand when a test for it is requisitioned, the lab can get away with using a Lyme disease test kit instead. The chances of cross-reactivity are so high that a Lyme test will likely return a positive result in the presence of antibodies to the relapsing tick fever bacterium. It's the patient's symptoms and risk exposure that will then tip the scales when doctors are considering which illness is really at play.

Indeed, BC researchers have long expressed concerns over specificity issues surrounding the tests for relapsing tick fever and until the past decade, the Provincial Laboratory at the British Columbia Centre for Disease Control was marking test results for relapsing tick fever as "investigational" in an effort to caution doctors against relying on them too heavily in diagnostic situations. (That's no longer the case.)

The problem, of course, is that doctors would need to have enough clinical experience with both diseases in order to be able to distinguish between them in the absence of conclusive test results; otherwise, they have no choice but to guess.

And in Canada, where Lyme is considered to be a rare disease and relapsing tick fever is considered to be an extremely rare disease, guessing rules the day.

I pass my hand in front of my eyes and watch as white trails streak out behind it then slowly dissolve. I can do this with either hand, but my central nervous system has decided to delist my left arm for the time being, so there's no point in even trying to move it until the nerves switch back on. I'd have a better chance of telepathically moving the dining room table to the roof.

Come to think of it, that could be an interesting way to blow a few hours. Maybe later.

I'm determined to stay focused on the trails streaking out behind my hand. These streaks are composed of countless replicas of my own arm, all hewn from translucent white light and all overlapping, so that when I sweep my arm in front of my eyes I see something akin to a courtesan's fan splaying open then slowly dissolving. The fan effect happens if I move my arm in front of my face when the lighting is dim.

Anything else can move past me — or I past it — and no trails appear. I have yet to figure out why this is. Maybe it's a distance thing and my arm is exactly the right distance from my eyes to trigger the effect. Or maybe my brain can't initiate an arm movement and track it visually unless the lights are fully ablaze. Or maybe the trails are there all the time and I just don't notice them when the lighting is bright or when something other than my arm passes close.

Maybe can lead me to some interesting places.

So can my brain. It can clone the objects around me in white light, showing me the object as it truly exists slightly offset from its translucent white twin, much like a drop-shadow or, more accurately, a drop-highlight. As with the arm-trails, this oddity only occurs in dim light.

It's also inconsistent. Sometimes the translucent twin is visible, sometimes it isn't. What determines when the effect appears remains a mystery. But when it does show up, it shows up abruptly, causing me to jerk to one side to avoid colliding with the edge of an object that's suddenly jutting towards me. It's only after I react that I realize what I'm trying to avoid is a phantom.

HUBRIS NEVER SLEEPS

There's a book with a bright white spine on a shelf in my library. It often catches my eye as I shuffle past, but reading is difficult these days. It would be easier for me to decipher a parchment written in some long-forgotten language than for me to read a single paragraph written in my native tongue.

Today, however, I'm bored and I'm restless and I'm up for the challenge of doing something that will give me that rare feeling of normalcy, so I snap the book from its shelf and flip it open to the page I long ago flagged with a bookmark.

It takes a few moments for me to recognize any words. My eyes slide aimlessly over the page like a dog on slick ice, not able to gain traction against the odd symbols that refuse to resolve into language until finally I force myself to remember the rules they taught me in grade school.

I train my eyes on the top left of the page and nail a word down. Then I nail down another.

I sound out each syllable as I encounter it, thinking that if I can just hear how a word sounds then somehow it will become fixed in my mind. And so it does.

The bookmark becomes my assistant. I use it to underscore each line as I fumble from left to right. If I don't do this, my eyes slip off the end of the line and are unable to find their way to the beginning of the next one.

In this way I build sentences.

The subject of the book I'm attempting to read is the deer proofing of gardens. For those of us who dare to grow vegetables on rural properties, the information contained between its covers can mean the difference between feast and famine.

I set this book aside a few years ago when I discovered that I wasn't able to process any of the advice it was giving. I told myself that was because the book was so boring that my brain was rejecting the words without acknowledging their right to exist.

It was the easy thing to believe. It protected me from admitting that something had gone terribly wrong in my brain. And I needed to be protected from that, so I carried the book around with me for a long time after I could no longer puzzle out the meanings behind its words. The bookmark never advanced, but as long as the book was at my fingertips, the possibility remained that it could advance just as soon as whatever was wrong with me passed. Only it didn't pass.

So here I am all these years later and once again I'm determined to learn a thing or two about protecting my squash from marauding deer.

Only I've hit a snag. The page the bookmark has so valiantly flagged all this time deals with a disease that can ravage humans when they share space with deer. Specifically, the bookmark is flagging the page on Lyme disease.

At first I think my brain is playing a trick on me. It does that. My brain has developed a cruel sense of humor.

But no, the page I bookmarked so long ago gives an overview of the disease that's implicated in the destruction of life as I once knew it.

This sends a chill down my spine.

If someone were to ask me, I would say that the first time I became aware that Lyme disease was the illness that fractured my mind was when I received the phone call from the dude who might sweep the floors at the public health department. I hadn't known until that moment that Lyme had been a possibility. It wasn't one of the diseases that doctors had paraded before me. I didn't even know I'd been tested for it. So the news came as something of a shock.

Or did it? One part of my brain is inclined to believe that the placement of the bookmark is just a coincidence. I stopped reading the book at that point because that's where frustration surpassed curiosity. Another part of my brain is inclined to believe something quite different. It insists that I stopped reading at that point because the name of my disease resonated somewhere deep inside my subconscious. And that resonance so disturbed me that I couldn't bear to read another word. There's no way for me to know which part of my brain is correct. I have no idea what I knew — or even what I suspected — back then.

On a conscious level, I don't believe Lyme registered until the day of that fateful phone call. But there's far more to human experience than what registers on a conscious level and I'm inclined to believe that maybe the nagging part of my brain is correct, that something deep inside of me knew all along what was wrong and tried in vain to convey that knowledge to a part of my brain that could act on it.

And I responded by closing the book.

Hubris, it seems, never sleeps.

The one positive thing about being diagnosed with both Lyme disease and relapsing tick fever is that it's become something of a litmus test. Stating my diagnosis allows me to instantly and effortlessly determine how well the person I'm talking to knows their tick-borne illnesses. There should be a reaction to the diagnosis. A raised eyebrow. An awkward silence. A confused grin. Something, anything, to tell me that the person I'm speaking to knows just how odd that diagnosis is.

Not one medical doctor has ever expressed surprise.

Not one Lyme researcher has failed to express it. Each researcher I contacted stated pretty much the same thing: They had never heard of one person being diagnosed with both illnesses. Indeed, my own research mostly confirms what they were telling me. Mostly.

I did, however, manage to track down a paper acknowledging that there appears to be a rare group of people on this continent showing signs of having both illnesses. That paper describes three patients who share my predicament. Those patients are variously located in northern California, Alberta, and my home province of British Columbia. All under the western flight path of migratory birds.

Maybe that's a coincidence. Maybe it's significant. Maybe someday someone will provide the missing piece to this puzzle. Because it surely is a puzzle.

But considering there's so little data linking the two illnesses, I'm guessing that someday won't be arriving any time soon.

That I received different results on the Western blots for Bb and Bh may ultimately not be meaningful. That discrepancy may simply underline a reproducibility issue that has long dogged borrelia testing. It's possible that if I'd had two sets of Lyme tests or two sets of relapsing tick fever tests instead of one of each, I still would've received two different results.

If labs have trouble reproducing test results when identical tests are run on identical samples — something that's been shown to be the case — then there's no reason to believe they'll be any more accurate when running those same tests on two different samples taken on two different days, even if they come from the same patient. A lot can change in the space of a few days, especially when you're dealing with fevers that magically appear, disappear, then reappear.

So let's focus on the fevers for a moment. During episodes of scorching hot fevers, someone suffering from relapsing tick fever can develop a condition known as spirochetemia — a fancy word that means there's a sudden, dramatic increase in the amount of borrelia bacteria in the body — which the immune system immediately counteracts with a correspondingly dramatic increase in the number of antibodies to that bacteria.

Since the tests for both Lyme disease and relapsing tick fever are antibody tests, blood drawn during or just after a fever episode will likely contain many more antibodies than blood drawn during an afebrile period, potentially affecting test results. Remember, one of the problems with the Lyme tests is that there are often too few antibodies present in a sample for those tests to be effective. That problem doesn't exist when spirochetemia is in play.

There should be more than enough antibodies present to trigger a positive test for Lyme disease even if the underlying bacterium is a species of borrelia that causes relapsing tick fever. And a positive test is exactly what I got.

The opposite is also true. A test done on blood that's been taken during an afebrile period can reasonably be expected to come back negative on an antibody test for borrelia bacteria, regardless of whether the test is for Lyme disease or relapsing tick fever due to the low number of antibodies present. It wouldn't be the first time. Far from it.

So maybe I should consider myself lucky. Had my fevers not been present, relapsing tick fever — the illness that was originally clinically diagnosed, subsequently dumped based on a positive Lyme test, then brought back into the diagnosis when no other explanation could be found for those distinctive fevers — would've been removed as a possible cause of my troubles, all thanks to the results of some flawed tests, which appeared to rule it out. And Lyme disease — a disease for which low antibody response often causes tests to come back negative — might very well never have been diagnosed, something that would no doubt have caused the one disease on so many doctors' lips — multiple sclerosis — to be my diagnostic fate.

The funny thing is — and if you're me, it's really quite hilarious — even though I've been diagnosed with an ironclad case of Lyme disease that no public health official or medical doctor has dared to overturn (one of just a handful of people each year nationwide to be counted in the official Lyme statistics), I may never have had that disease at all.

✳

My official diagnosis says that at some point (or maybe a couple of different points) in my life I became infected with both Lyme disease and relapsing tick fever.

My official diagnosis is ridiculous.

That doesn't mean it isn't accurate, it just means that when anyone who knows anything about Lyme disease asks me if I've been diagnosed with one of its co-infections I hesitate before answering.

Technically the answer is no.

I haven't been diagnosed with one of Lyme's co-infections.

Relapsing tick fever isn't one of Lyme's co-infections.

Without a common vector, the two illnesses can't infect the same individual.

At least, not easily.

I'd have a better chance of being struck by lightning, attacked by a cougar, and thrown off a building — all on the same day — than to contract those two illnesses in the space of a single lifetime.

There are days when I feel like I have been.

If I'm feeling brave enough to admit what my diagnosis is to someone who is actually knowledgeable about tick-borne illnesses, my bravery is typically greeted with confusion, disbelief or surprise.

Rarely is it greeted with silence.

I've been asked — not impolitely — if a medical doctor gave me that diagnosis or if I diagnosed myself. And I understand where the question is coming from. No one can quite believe that a doctor would inflict such an odd diagnosis on me.

I can't quite believe it myself.

So mostly I don't admit what my diagnosis is.

Mostly I stay silent.

I'm not entirely certain whom that silence is designed to protect.

✳

There's a saying in the medical profession that goes something like this: If you hear hoof beats, don't think zebra.

I think the sentiment is obvious.

If a patient walks into a doctor's office with symptoms that can be ascribed to two illnesses, one common, the other rare, that patient most likely has the common illness. The rest of the scientific world knows this principle as Occam's Razor, which states that when two possible explanations exist for the presence of a phenomenon, the simplest explanation is most likely the correct one.

But the rest of the scientific world doesn't concern me right now.

I've been diagnosed with a zebra.

Maybe I've been diagnosed as a zebra.

You could even make the case that I've been diagnosed as a zebra with horizontal and vertical stripes, since both illnesses are rare enough that having one would be unique in its own right, but both together is a bit outlandish.

Not that I'm above doing something that's a bit outlandish.

I suppose I should accept that and embrace my inner zebra. But before I do, there's a question I need to ask — a fairly obvious one — and that question is this: Is there a simpler explanation for the fevers? For instance, could they be the result of infection with an oddball strain of Bb? With literally hundreds of identified strains, it's hard to believe that researchers can definitively state every symptom caused by every strain of a bacterium that's only been known to exist for thirty years. There hasn't been enough time to conduct all that research, so it's conceivable that I was infected with one of the lesser-known (or unknown) strains of Bb, which just happens to cause a remitting/recurring fever more typical of relapsing tick fever.

Or what about this: You'll remember I noted earlier that babesia is found in the same ticks as Lyme disease and that of all Lyme's co-infections, it's by far the most common. It causes malarial fevers and a clinical picture that's both more severe and longer in duration than when Lyme arrives alone. Since it can hardly be argued that I have a mild case of Lyme or even one that's been short in duration, and since babesia infections do occur in British Columbia, then why not babesia?

I was tested for that disease and those tests came back negative.

But those tests are no more definitive than Lyme tests are. False negatives are common due to many factors, including the strains of babesia being tested for, the timing of the tests, the severity of the infection, and whether or not a fever was present when the blood was drawn. These problems are so well-documented that tests for babesia are performed multiple times on multiple samples taken on different days from a single patient in an effort to minimize false negatives.

Wrap your brain around that one.

So I can only cross my fingers and hope against hope that the results I received were accurate.

I don't have much choice.

Hoping against hope rules the day when it comes to testing for tick-borne illnesses and when it comes to babesia, testing is all we have. Getting an accurate clinical diagnosis was never a realistic possibility. Most doctors I talked to didn't even know what babesiosis was, let alone have the capacity to diagnose it.

The answer to my problem clearly wasn't going to be found in a doctor's office. And although I've explored many avenues looking for a simple explanation for the symptoms continuing to haunt me, I keep drawing blanks. Possibilities exist, to be sure, but somehow they never quite pan out. The diagnosis of relapsing tick fever and Lyme disease, improbable though it may be, remains the only explanation that covers all the bases.

And yet.

For the longest time I persisted in believing that something was going to happen to prove my diagnosis wrong. A kidney would fail or a new test would be developed or angels would float down from the clouds and sing the answer into being.

Who knows what I was waiting for.

I just felt that if I was patient and kept my eyes open, sooner or later the answer would arrive. And the answer did arrive. It just wasn't the answer I thought I was expecting. You see, I have a vivid memory of being told by one well-meaning researcher that I couldn't be suffering from the effects of both Lyme disease and relapsing tick fever because they don't share a common vector. This is something that each subsequent researcher I contacted agreed upon and, to be fair, all I had to do was read research papers on these two illnesses to see for myself that different ticks are named as vectors for the two diseases. So if I'd defied the odds and contracted both illnesses, I must necessarily have been bitten by two different ticks, possibly months, years, or even decades apart. It was a remote possibility, absolutely, but it was a logical one.

There was consensus on this point.

And consensus is a rare thing where Lyme disease is concerned, so when it puts in one of its infrequent appearances, it stands out like a solar eclipse.

But something interesting happened on the way to certitude.

In 2010, Canadian researchers decided to study *Ixodes scapularis* ticks collected from multiple sites stretching from Alberta to Nova Scotia in an effort to determine if the genetic diversity of Bb might be playing a role in the accuracy (or rather the inaccuracy) of diagnostic testing in this country.

That's when they discovered something quite unexpected.

They found relapsing tick fever borrelia and Lyme borrelia living side-by-side in the guts of some of those ticks. It was a landmark finding because it meant that for the first time proof had been found in nature that a person living in Canada could contract both illnesses from the bite of a single tick. It also meant that my diagnosis was suddenly not as improbable as it first appeared. I really could have contracted both relapsing tick fever and Lyme disease from one tick; the proof of that was sitting in government research facilities.

And not just in 2007, either. Technically, infection with both illnesses has been possible in this country for quite some time. The ticks used in the 2010 study had been collected as far back as 2005, and who knows how many years previous to that ticks had been carrying dual infections without anybody noticing?

That's anyone's guess.

Let's face it, unless you're looking for a needle in a haystack, you have no hope of finding one. Even when you're looking for one, it's pretty hard to spot one. So the fact that the researchers found the proof in the limited sample of ticks collected from across the country is really quite extraordinary.

Yet that's not the most interesting part of this anecdote.

The most interesting part is the species of relapsing tick fever borrelia living cheek by jowl with Bb in the guts of some of those ticks was not Bh, the species of relapsing tick fever that was presumed to have infected me, but rather a closely related "sister" species called *Borrelia miyamotoi*.

B. miyamotoi has an interesting history.

It was first discovered in Japan in the mid-1990s and although it was initially thought to make its home only in that country, it has since been found in other temperate regions, including Russia, the United States and now, belatedly, Canada. Indeed, in the northeastern United States, it's now estimated that *B. miyamotoi* accounts for up to 15 percent of the spirochetes carried by *I. scapularis* ticks. Not surprisingly, the bacterium has been found in the same white-footed mice that host Bb, firmly establishing its presence in nature in the United States.

No wonder it was found in Canadian ticks.

If Bb is moving from south to north — and it is — then why wouldn't other forms of borrelia be doing the same? They would, that's the point. When the ticks that carry these diseases move north, they necessarily bring with them any diseases they're carrying.

Logic doesn't get any simpler than that.

Initial research appears to suggest that a much lower percentage of the ticks in Canada are co-infected with Bb and *B. miyamatoi* than those in the United States, but keep in mind that initial research is all we have. Time will tell just how prevalent these co-infections are and also if *B. miyamotoi* is occurring in ticks in the absence of Bb, something that these first researchers couldn't report on because they weren't actually looking for *B. miyamotoi* at the time they discovered it. They were cataloguing different strains of Bb and, as a result, the only *B. miyamotoi* specimens they know about are the ones that occurred in tandem with the Bb bacterium they were targeting.

It does, however, seem likely that *B. miyamotoi* is occurring in ticks in the absence of Bb. It would be strange if it wasn't.

Part of what makes *B. miyamotoi* so interesting is that its symptoms can span those of both Lyme disease and relapsing tick fever. There's even some evidence to suggest that its clinical symptoms are both more diverse and more severe than those you'd expect to see in someone infected with Bb. Indeed, for some patients, a *B. miyamotoi* infection is a lot like having Lyme disease with the added bonus of the dramatic remitting/recurring fevers long associated with relapsing tick fever.

I'm sure you can see why the discovery of this particular species of borrelia in Canada caught my eye. I was tested for both relapsing tick fever and Lyme disease because I appeared to have the symptoms of both diseases and I lived in a region where both are endemic. At the time, no one considered that one species of borrelia could be causing the full range of symptoms because no single borrelia species had ever been discovered that was known to do that. And yet the specificity issues surrounding antibody testing make it entirely possible that a species of borrelia other than Bb or Bh could have been at the root of my illness. *B. miyamotoi* is just as much of a contender as any other.

What this means is that it's no longer necessary for me to have been bitten by two different ticks. I could've been bitten by a single tick carrying both illnesses or — more intriguingly — I could've been bitten by a tick carrying a single species of borrelia — possibly *B. miyamotoi,* possibly something else — which gave rise to the symptoms of both illnesses.

One of the interesting features of *B. miyamotoi* is that people who contract it often don't develop the distinctive EM rash that public health officials insist are common in Lyme infections.

Now there's something to contemplate.

It would go far towards explaining why I didn't develop such a rash.

Still, the discovery of *B. miyamotoi* in Canada (or anywhere else, for that matter) isn't really all that surprising. Research into borrelia bacteria is in its infancy worldwide. In the last decade, several new species have been discovered and although researchers don't know how many more they have yet to find, the one thing they're certain of is they will be finding more. There are lots of different types of borrelia bacteria out there and the process of cataloguing them all will span many decades to come.

It's intriguing to think that twenty years ago, no one had ever heard of *Borrelia lonestari, Borrelia theileri,* or *Borrelia miyamotoi,* but they have all since been discovered in the guts of ticks and given names. There are also other novel borrelia species that have been discovered in recent years and are still so new that their official names have yet to be established and, in some cases, the ticks that are vectoring these species into mammals remain unknown.

No one knows at this point what role (if any) many of these species play in human infection.

Those answers are still to come.

And here's something to contemplate: The three species of borrelia I've just listed above by name were all found in the guts of ixodid ticks — the hard-bodied ticks that carry Lyme disease — and yet all three are types of borrelia associated with relapsing tick fever, which is supposed to be carried by soft-bodied argasid ticks.

That's what the textbooks say.

That's the assumption researchers had been operating under.

These discoveries are problematic for several reasons. For one, if assumptions over which types of ticks carry which type of borrelia bacteria prove to be only partially accurate, then what other assumptions are being made by researchers that are also only partially accurate or, for that matter, not accurate at all but based on accepted reasoning that has yet to be disproven?

That answer is still on the horizon.

These discoveries also mean that there may be borrelia infections occurring in Canada for which no diagnostic tests currently exist. After all, tests have only been developed for a few species of borrelia and those tests are problematic at the best of times. Using them to detect borrelia species or even strains of Bb not previously known to exist — or worse, to identify multiple species of borrelia in a single person — is something they simply weren't designed to do. It'll likely be many years and require significant technological advancements before the tests that can accomplish these things are developed.

How does any of this help me?

Other than confirming that I could've contracted both illnesses from a single tick bite or possibly even have contracted a single bacterium whose symptoms span both illnesses, it doesn't help a whole lot. All anyone can say for certain is that somewhere along the line I became infected with at least one form of borrelia bacteria. There's no way for current diagnostic testing to say with any authority which form or even if the borrelia infecting me is a previously identified species or something new to science. That kind of specific diagnostic testing likely won't exist for many years.

Possibly even decades.

And it's questionable what use it'll be to me once it arrives since so much time will have passed — so much time has already passed — between infection and identification.

THE PERFECT HOST

Not one doctor I've seen since 2007 ever actually bothered to look up relapsing tick fever, from what I could tell. As far as they're concerned, that illness is a relic in my medical file that's no more or less interesting than the chicken pox I had as a child. The antibiotics I took in the summer of 2007 should've more than wiped out the infection.

And yet one day when I was looking up information on Lyme disease in a mostly futile effort to fill in a gap in knowledge that doctors had no interest in filling for me, I stumbled across something unexpected which, admittedly, is par for the course when it comes to researching borrelia infections.

What I stumbled across was a slide presentation on biofilms put together by some gung-ho Lyme researcher who was determined to show photographic evidence for each and every one of Bb's known survival forms, including the biofilms that were the presentation's primary focus.

There were a lot of slides. They showed biofilms, blebs, and cysts. They showed cell-wall deficient rebels. They even showed combinations of two or more survival forms. There was nothing in this presentation I hadn't seen before. I was seriously considering nodding off.

That's when I noticed the unexpected thing. One of the slides showed what appeared to be a microscopic image of a solitary Bb bacterium at the moment it was losing its cell wall, but the slide wasn't labeled Bb, it was labeled Bh — relapsing tick fever. A few slides later, there was that label again, beneath a different survival form.

It didn't really register at first. It kind of hit my brain and bounced, only to catch me on the rebound.

Relapsing tick fever and Lyme disease are closely related members of the same genus of bacteria and they both share a propensity for antigenic variation (albeit using slightly different mechanisms), so then why did it surprise me to discover that they also share a propensity for creating survival forms?

That set me on different track entirely.

It's amazing how easy it is to find something when you know what it is you're looking for. And what I was looking for was confirmation that relapsing tick fever can survive a supposedly lethal blast of antibiotics and live on as a chronic infection similar to Lyme disease. After all, survival forms are often blamed for Lyme's almost otherworldly ability to survive everything that's thrown at it, resulting in a slow-simmering illness that can last for months or even years after initial infection, assuming it's even curable, and no one has quite convinced me that it is. So if Lyme can survive the unsurvivable, what's stopping relapsing tick fever from doing the same thing?

Researchers have indeed shown that relapsing tick fever patients treated with antibiotics can go on to suffer symptoms of what appears to be a residual infection. In some cases, multiple courses of oral antibiotics have been given for as long as ten days at a shot and still they failed to halt the progress of the disease. In other cases, intravenous antibiotics were tried and again symptoms persisted.

The longer treatment was delayed after the first fever episode, the greater the chances that relapsing tick fever would linger. Just a few weeks' delay was enough for evidence of persistence to rear its ugly head. In my case, treatment was delayed more than five months, which my Spidey sense tells me was probably not a good thing.

The good news is that most people eventually recover from relapsing tick fever. The bad news, of course, is that a minority goes on to develop a chronic illness that they just can't seem to shake. That illness is known as chronic borreliosis and can cause all the same symptoms as chronic Lyme disease (which is technically known as Lyme borreliosis, for those of you who care about such things). The difference between the two illnesses is seen mainly in the first stage when relapsing tick fever earns its name. Once relapsing tick fever becomes chronic, its namesake symptom can vanish, mercifully freeing the patient from those raucous fever episodes, and yet the illness tends not to lose its relapsing nature.

This would certainly explain a few things. Like why I seem to go for long stretches during which my overall health seems to improve until one day, without warning, symptoms come roaring back seemingly from nowhere — a body blow from another dimension — and take me down hard. Those symptoms can affect any part of my body from my toes to my brain before slowly subsiding over the course of several weeks only to return again at a later date.

The ongoing cyclical nature of chronic borreliosis goes far towards explaining why these symptoms behave the way they do; why I often feel like a ribbon attached to the tailfin of some hulking, invisible leviathan that surfaces in a flurry of frenetic activity, then slips back silently under the waves until the urge to surface once again proves irresistible.

I wonder what it will take to pull myself free.

Or to hold the hulking beast underwater long enough to drown it.

When I was tested for both Lyme disease and relapsing tick fever way back in 2007, the tests were reactive with the IgG, but not the IgM, antibodies. I was told those results meant that I'd been exposed to Lyme at some point in my life, but that the disease was no longer active at the time the blood was drawn. Ditto for relapsing tick fever, except the test results for that disease were weaker, so the infection was likely even farther in my past.

It was an odd thing to be told. I mean, the blood for these tests was drawn while I was hospitalized for an acute illness that included remitting/recurring fevers that were like nothing I'd ever experienced before.

Unique in the world of illness, the experts say.

No kidding.

What doctors were asking me to believe was that during a span of time when I was being assailed by these fevers, vomiting my guts out, delirious as all get out, and every other symptom I described earlier in this book, there was no active infection. The distinctive relapsing fevers had nothing to do with an active relapsing tick fever infection (or even an active Lyme infection), but instead were due to...

I have no clue how to finish that sentence.

What doctors were telling me back then struck me as ridiculous. It still strikes me that way. It also wasn't true.

Neither the screening test nor the Western blot is capable of distinguishing between a previous or an ongoing borrelia infection. That doctors were telling me otherwise required they ignore the clinical evidence before them.

That I was actively battling an illness while I was in the hospital is without a doubt. Even a first-year medical student could've figured that bit out. A borrelia infection of some description (or possibly several) was still in there, switching up surface proteins in ever more inventive combinations so that my immune system would give up trying to knock it out, realize it'd been outsmarted, renew its attack, then break it off again in a seemingly inexhaustible display of fortitude against a diabolical foe wearing an endless array of disguises.

Suspension of disbelief is required when listening to so-called experts talk about Lyme disease.

There are those out there who disagree that the symptoms continuing to haunt me are the result of a persistent borrelia infection, something that seems obvious to me.

Over the years, I've been given a plethora of reasons for why I'm still exhibiting symptoms long after being diagnosed and treated for a borrelia infection. I've been told, for instance, that I'm suffering from the impressive-sounding Post-Lyme Disease Syndrome. This syndrome was cooked up as a way to explain why some Lyme patients continue to have symptoms after they've been treated with a short course of antibiotics. It can't be due to an ongoing infection with an antibiotic-resistant pathogen that's exceedingly difficult for existing tests to detect, so it must be due to something else.

That something else is Post-Lyme Disease Syndrome. The theory behind this syndrome is that Bb gets the immune system all riled up while it's present and even though the bacteria itself may have been defeated, the immune system continues to behave as though it hasn't been. Instead of breaking off the attack, it keeps trying to hunt down and destroy the invading bacteria that it can't quite believe aren't there anymore, causing all sorts of problems that make it seem like someone is still battling an active infection when really they aren't. That's the gist of it, anyway.

According to the syndrome theory of ongoing symptoms, once my immune system stops being so reactionary, things will calm down. Someday. Possibly before I die. No guarantees on that one. That's one theory.

I've also been told that the sorts of ongoing neurological problems that have been plaguing me are a known outcome for a minority of Lyme patients. The jury is still out on why this happens, but prolonged antibiotic treatment seems to have little effect. Maybe the symptoms will subside over time. Maybe they won't.

They're not necessarily the result of a syndrome, but no one can say for certain what they're the result of. Possibly a tick-borne infection that's still unknown to medical science — a prion maybe, or a virus. Whatever it is, antibiotics don't seem to touch it.

Then there's the theory that at some point during the worst of my illness I suffered diffuse nerve and brain damage, possibly as a result of the catastrophically high fevers, possibly as a result of restricted blood flow in my brain, possibly as a result of severe, persistent inflammation just about everywhere, or possibly as a result of healthy cells being damaged by a panicking immune system. Whatever. This hypothesized damage doesn't show up on an MRI, so it's hard for me to invest a whole lot of confidence in this theory.

Then there's the suggestion that at least some of my symptoms may be the result of abnormal electrical activity in my brain — what normal people call seizures — but that too has never been conclusively proven.

And there's yet another theory that my symptoms are psychosomatic and will go away as soon as I ditch the crazy. This theory amuses me to no end. Talk about not putting the effort in.

I don't find any of these theories particularly helpful since they never result in actionable conclusions. Indeed, their only purpose, as far as I can make out, is to let doctors off the hook for doing anything useful to help me.

And always I think: Occam's Razor. If the simplest explanation for a problem is most often the correct one, then wouldn't the simplest explanation for why someone who has been treated for an infection continues to experience the symptoms associated with that infection be that the treatment failed and the infection is still active?

Of course, this explanation means that we're dealing with an antibiotic-resistant stealth infection for which effective treatment may not even have been invented, but the basic problem here is that any other explanation requires proof beyond mere gut instinct and no one has yet been able to pony up that proof.

Nor can I prove that any of these diverse theories are wrong.

That, in a nutshell, is the reason why a principle such as Occam's Razor exists. It's a principle that essentially says that if you find yourself in a situation where you have no choice but to guess, keep it simple. The most obvious answer is likely the correct one. And the most obvious reason why my symptoms didn't magically cease in the wake of antibiotic treatment is that those antibiotics did not eradicate the infection.

THE RULES OF ENGAGEMENT

I'm sitting in a doctor's office for some reason that has nothing whatsoever to do with Lyme disease. I long ago stopped talking to doctors about Lyme They refuse to believe that a short course of antibiotics failed to eradicate the illness and I refuse to be treated like a pariah.

The rules of engagement have been clearly defined.

But the appointment is a struggle. I'm confused and mildly disoriented and I'm sure I'm acting strangely. I'm certainly thinking strangely. I blurt out responses that make little sense, even to me, and mostly I wish I could take control of my mouth so that it'll stop saying stupid things.

The doctor pauses.

He suggests, without any sort of verbal foreplay, that I might want to consider going on long-term antibiotics. Not that he's willing to write the prescription himself, mind you. No, it seems going toe-to-toe with a disciplinary committee at The College isn't his thing.

But he knows a guy.

Presumably another doctor, but I don't inquire and he doesn't volunteer.

He's testing the water in much the same way a doctor in the 1950s might bring up the topic of a back-alley abortion to see what sort of reaction he gets before plunging in.

He's also looking down at his desk as he speaks. Or maybe it's the back of his hands he's looking at. What he isn't looking at is me. Pointedly.

But I'm certainly looking at him.

There's one thought cycling through my mind: Treatment delayed is treatment denied. This conversation should've happened when I was first diagnosed with Lyme. This conversation *did* happen when I was first diagnosed with Lyme and it went nowhere because the only doctor willing to treat me with antibiotics beyond a month was being investigated by The College. No other doctor was willing to even acknowledge that treating Lyme beyond a month was an option.

Then. And then is all that really matters.

I'm not willing to have this conversation now with a doctor who so clearly feels compromised by his own suggestion. It's like trying to talk about sex with your parents, and really, it shouldn't be. This should be a dispassionate discussion about medical treatment, not a moral dilemma. But a moral dilemma is clearly what the doctor is feeling and I don't have the heart to tell him that if I'm going to do something radical, it won't be with the help of some dilettante doctor with little experience in defying authority. No, it'll be with the help of someone for whom defiance of authority has become habitual.

Someone not under the thumb of The College.

Someone this doctor has never met.

This is really what I think.

Maybe I should explain why this doctor was feeling so conflicted; why he didn't just whip out his prescription pad and administer the treatment that he had slowly come to realize might bring me some relief, if not an all-out cure.

Two sets of treatment guidelines exert tremendous influence on how Lyme disease is handled in both Canada and the United States.

The first set is put out by the Infectious Disease Society of America (IDSA) and narrowly defines Lyme as infection with Bb. These guidelines don't recognize any other species of borrelia as being causative, nor do they mention any ticks other than *Ixodes scapularis* and *Ixodes pacificus* as carriers of the Lyme bacteria.

It's indeed an orderly world in which these authors operate.

The IDSA guidelines recognize just two legitimate categories of Lyme infections: Early and late. Anyone suffering from an early infection can, according to the authors, reasonably expect to be cured by popping oral antibiotics for a period of between two weeks and a month.

Unless, that is, there are clear signs of a neurological infection.

For those patients whose brains are melting down, intravenous antibiotics are the way to go, but again, one month is the maximum recommended duration for such treatment. In the rare event that symptoms outlast the antibiotics, another round can be considered.

But it's best not to make a habit of it.

The authors of the IDSA guidelines can find no compelling evidence that chronic Lyme disease infections exist and instead suggest that ongoing symptoms are most likely the result of Post-Lyme Disease Syndrome. Symptoms may also be the result of a co-infection with other tick-borne organisms, previously undiagnosed autoimmune ailments, or psychological problems. The authors dismiss the idea that a prolonged infection with Lyme bacteria could be at the root of these ongoing symptoms and don't believe that the use of long-term antibiotics has any significant effect on the outcome of the disease.

The second set of guidelines is put out by the International Lyme and Associated Diseases Society (ILADS). These guidelines recognize three categories of infection: Early localized, Disseminated, and Chronic. They go on to make the case for Lyme disease being an antibiotic-resistant stealth infection that often calls for prolonged courses of treatment using combinations of different classes of antibiotics. Indeed, the majority of the ILADS guidelines focus on how to deal with just the sort of chronic Lyme infections that the authors of the IDSA guidelines dismiss. Not surprisingly, the ILADS guidelines dismiss Post-Lyme Disease Syndrome, making the case that ongoing symptoms — particularly those that are neurological or arthritic in nature — are more likely the result of ongoing infection.

Both of these guidelines are highly influential. Both are considered to be the gold standard for Lyme treatment by those who adhere to them.

However, mainstream medical practice in both the United States and Canada has embraced the IDSA guidelines, which means that anyone in either country whose symptoms outlast one month of antibiotic treatment is considered by default to be suffering from a syndrome that requires no treatment beyond that which has already been given.

It doesn't matter that a conflicting set of guidelines exists.

And it doesn't matter what the patients themselves think. Those patients in Canada who are convinced that the antibiotic treatment they received failed to cure them find themselves in the position of trying to locate a doctor willing to break with mainstream medicine to treat Lyme according to the tenets of the ILADS guidelines.

Good luck with that. Those doctors exist, but they're few and far between. And they're difficult to find. Their names are never spoken publically. Only in whispers. On notes passed in darkened rooms. By a doctor who knows a guy.

This isn't done to protect the doctors who are treating Lyme in defiance of the IDSA guidelines. No, it is done to protect Lyme patients, who will have nowhere left to turn if health authorities decide to go after those few doctors willing to treat patients beyond 30 days. It's not like it hasn't happened before. It happened in British Columbia and everyone knows it.

So the names of doctors willing to treat Lyme are passed around in secrecy, without anyone telling the authorities that it's happening.

Is this really how medicine is practiced in Canada? Yes, it really is. How far we've fallen.

When I was diagnosed with Lyme disease way back in 2007, just 12 other people in British Columbia shared the dubious distinction of having their cases of Lyme officially confirmed by those who have the power to officially confirm such things.

And that was a banner year. Normally, there are roughly half that many confirmed cases in the province annually, a rate that has remained stable for more than a decade. Those cases come to the attention of public health authorities through several sources, including laboratory results, surveillance data, and reporting by doctors.

Doctors and public health employees alike told me I was suffering from an illness that's considered rare both in this province and across the country. Indeed, if only 13 people in a province just shy of 4.5 million residents comes down with an illness, it would be hard to argue that an epidemic is underway.

And yet, from the beginning, something didn't sit right. The more people I mentioned Lyme to, the more people I discovered who either had the illness themselves or knew of someone who did. There seemed to be whole lot more Lyme sufferers than official statistics accounted for. There seemed to be legions.

Lyme disease was a reportable illness in British Columbia when I was diagnosed with it in 2007 (it became nationally reportable in 2009), which means that when someone is diagnosed with the illness, the doctor who made that diagnosis is legally obligated to report it to public health authorities. (Although public health authorities knew my diagnosis before my doctor did, so the lab must have reported me before my doctor had the chance.)

But were doctors really doing what they were supposed to?

In 2008, the BC Centre for Disease Control and the College of Physicians and Surgeons of BC got together and sent a voluntary survey to the BC doctors they deemed most likely to run across Lyme — pediatricians, internists, and family practitioners among them — in an effort to determine how well these doctors knew Lyme and to see if any of them had diagnosed any cases of the disease during the previous calendar year.

The results were intriguing. Just over 30 percent of doctors who received the survey responded to it, but those who did copped to diagnosing 221 cases of Lyme disease in 2007 alone.

And those are just the cases that the target doctors knew about. They don't include those patients who left the healthcare system to get their disease diagnosed and treated in another country and were too angry or exasperated to inform their doctors in BC. They also don't include patients who were (or possibly still are) under the impression that multiple sclerosis or lupus or any one of the dozens of autoimmune illnesses that Lyme is commonly mistaken for is the cause of their misery. Nor do they include those patients who haven't yet received a diagnosis of any kind, but who are busy being swatted around a healthcare system that doesn't know what to do with symptoms that don't fit neatly inside diagnostic boxes. And they certainly don't include any cases diagnosed by doctors not targeted by the survey.

In short, the cases reported on this survey don't include a whole lot of people.

Yet there's a notable chasm between the numbers of official Lyme cases and the number truly diagnosed. The discrepancy between the 13 officially logged cases and the 221 cases reported by doctors in this survey is certainly striking. I wouldn't have expected the numbers to be identical, but I would've expected them to be closer than that. Then again, it's estimated the true number of Lyme cases in the United States each year is between ten and twenty times the figures put out by the Center for Disease Control in Atlanta due to underreporting by doctors. So it seems that British Columbia's doctors are no lazier than their American counterparts when it comes to fulfilling their reporting obligations.

What's more striking is that just over 30 percent of doctors returned their surveys. I can only imagine what the numbers would've been if 50 percent of doctors had responded or — gasp — 75 percent of them. We'll never know.

The one thing we do know is that Lyme disease — though not nearly as prevalent as the seasonal flu — isn't nearly as rare as I was led to believe, not by a long shot. But then I'd already figured that out on my own. I didn't need a survey to confirm what I was discovering all around me.

What I did need a survey to confirm was that more doctors were willing to report their Lyme cases on a voluntary survey they were in no way obligated to participate in than were willing to report them to public health authorities at the time of diagnosis even though they were legally obligated to do so. Significantly more.

Maybe the case definition of Lyme is so narrow that most people who suffer from Lyme disease don't fit the strict criteria used to define the illness. Maybe doctors knew that their patients would be on the receiving end of intrusive phone calls from public health employees and wanted to save them the hassle. Then again, maybe doctors don't think enough of public health authorities to clue them in on what's going on all around them.

Or maybe, just maybe, they couldn't be bothered.

Whatever the reasons doctors in BC didn't report their Lyme cases to the authorities when they were supposed to, the one thing it can't be blamed on is their ignorance regarding whether the illness was reportable. Roughly two-thirds of doctors surveyed admitted they did know that and yet most of them still didn't report their cases to the proper authorities as required by law.

It makes you wonder just what the sanctions for a doctor not complying with the compulsory obligation to report a disease are. I'm betting they aren't much. I'm also betting that few if any doctors have ever been sanctioned for non-reporting, proving that even doctors know a toothless tiger when they see one.

When taken on their own, the results of the survey are troubling. They become even more so when combined with the assertions by public health officials in British Columbia that more than 80 percent of all Lyme disease patients develop a distinctive EM rash.

How can they possibly know this?

If only 13 cases of the 221 that doctors diagnosed in 2007 were officially recorded, then how can public health officials state with any degree of accuracy that 80 percent of Lyme patients develop an EM rash when they weren't aware of 80 percent of the Lyme patients in this province in 2007?

They weren't even aware of six percent of the cases.

They were aware of 13 people.

(In the wake of the survey, a fourteenth person would be added to the official statistics.)

Until public health authorities track down those patients who weren't turned in to them in 2007 — something I'm thinking isn't likely to ever happen — they can't really make any definitive statements about what percentage of Lyme patients developed a rash that year or, for that matter, any other.

It's not like doctors are getting any better at reporting Lyme disease.

In 2008, six cases were recorded by the British Columbia Centre for Disease Control and in 2009, a whopping 10 cases were recorded.

But how many cases of Lyme were actually diagnosed?

Unless someone sends out another voluntary survey, it's unlikely we'll ever know the answer to that question. Logic says the number of infected people didn't magically drop from 221 in 2007 to six in 2008, so then what's the true number of Lyme cases diagnosed on average each year in this province? 180? 340? Something in between?

While trying to track down the answer to this question, I stumbled across an interesting phenomenon that occurred in one region of the United States between 1989 and 1991. Doctors in the state of Georgia reported 715 cases of Lyme to the CDC in Atlanta that first year, 161 cases the next, and just 28 cases in the third year.

Why the dramatic drop? Did Lyme pack up and move someplace more to its liking?

Well, it seems that the CDC took the position that there was no evidence of Lyme disease in nature in that state and therefore there could be no Lyme disease in human patients originating from Georgia, so the reported cases must be false. Doctors responded by refraining from reporting their Lyme cases to the CDC and everyone was happy.

Except possibly the patients.

There's a parallel in British Columbia where the BC CDC states, rather emphatically, that the infection rate in *Ixodes pacificus* ticks in this province is less than one percent, that these ticks are reluctant to bite humans, and that there are fewer than 0.5 cases per 100,000 people each year in BC.

Now that's a rare disease.

At least officially.

Any doctor who reports a case will be singling a patient out. They'll also be singling themselves out, especially if they report more than one case. And who wants to draw that sort of attention to themselves and risk being called a zealot, an incompetent, or worse? It's much less hassle to quietly diagnose and treat these cases without letting the authorities know they exist.

For everyone.

Enough about British Columbia. It's of interest to me because I live here, but maybe you live in Ontario or Manitoba or Nunavut. So how does the rest of Canada fare when it comes to Lyme reporting?

In 2006, the Public Health Agency of Canada (PHAC) held a meeting focusing on Lyme disease and concluded that, on average, there are between 20 and 60 new cases of Lyme disease each year nationwide. The number of confirmed cases in Canada has since been revised upwards, with an all-time high of 258 cases recorded in 2011.

Just like in British Columbia, Lyme is considered to be a rare disease nationwide. Assuming, of course, that the official numbers are even close to being accurate, and likely they aren't. The voluntary survey of BC doctors shows that more than 221 new cases of Lyme were diagnosed in British Columbia in one year alone, meaning that the numbers stated nationally must necessarily be on the low side since they barely account for the cases in a single province and Lyme disease doesn't occur in just one province. It occurs in all of them.

What interests me most about the claims of a government agency that just 258 people from across Canada each year are becoming infected with Lyme is that almost 13,000 confirmed cases (remember, you have to multiply that figure by at least ten to get the true number due to underreporting) are recorded each year in the ten states that share a border with Canadian provinces. It seems quite unlikely that only 258 new infections each year are occurring in this country, especially when you consider that the vast majority of Canadians live within 200 kilometers of the US border. Many of us have even crossed that border.

In light of all this, I find myself asking — and this is a sincere question — at what point do public health officials admit they don't actually know how many people in Canada are suffering from Lyme disease? Because it's clear they don't, and making like they do can't possibly be in the best interests of Canadians who are trying to keep themselves and their families healthy.

In 2009, two years after I took my case of Lyme out of the healthcare system for the first time, I relented somewhat, and returned to seek further assessment of my condition.

But then you already figured that out, didn't you?

My primary goal this time around was to satisfy myself that doctors really did know nothing about Lyme disease. I'd been so sick the first time around and so frustrated by how poorly I'd been treated that it was possible I hadn't given doctors a fair shake back when I was first diagnosed.

So I went back.

But doctors in 2009 were just as clueless as they were in 2007. When I asked pointed questions about my illness — because by then I knew which questions to ask — I was routinely greeted by unsubstantiated guesses, cultural biases, and information plagiarized from woefully inadequate sources, all of which were being passed off as medical expertise.

That tactic probably works if a patient hasn't taken the time to research her illness, but it fails miserably if she has. All it does is produce a twinge in the pit of her stomach; a twinge that tells her that once again it's time to leave before someone goes and does something stupid. And trusting the advice of medical doctors who don't even have the decency to acknowledge the limits of their knowledge tops the list of stupid things a person could do.

SHIFTING SANDS

When I read the many fragments of writing that form the basis of this book, I'm faced with the person I was when Lyme disease was at its worst; a person who existed in isolation, cut off from the world by pain and fear and symptoms that no one seemed able to understand.

Several of the passages in this book are artifacts with no memories attached.

As I read through them now, they seem like the words a prisoner might scratch into a cell wall hoping that someone, someday, might read them and know that in this place someone as real and as human as they are suffered.

I didn't think at the time that I would survive my battle with Lyme. Or, if I did survive it, that it would be without permanent damage; in that respect, I was correct.

I wish I could reach back through time — through the pain and the isolation and the fear — and take the person I was during those moments by the hand and tell her that it was all going to be okay. That she would survive the worst this disease could throw at her and come to a place of relative peace where Lyme and her spirit could share the same body, each having negotiated for a compromised right to survive.

If there's one thing that Lyme has taught me it's that fear is finite. There truly is only so afraid one person can get before the terror crescendos, then shatters and falls away. Now whenever my heart beats out a syncopated rhythm or my fingers turn gunmetal blue, panic fails to arrive. I watch and I wait, as curious as an economist about what will happen next and equally dispassionate about the outcome.

How things have changed.

I didn't know much about Lyme disease when it was playing roulette with my life, partly because the effects of the disease made it difficult for me to look things up and partly because there were no experts I could consult in a medical system that had chosen to turn a blind eye on a disease that it didn't want to have anything to do with. I've learned a lot about Lyme since then and have woven much of what I learned into this book, hoping to make sense of everything that happened, if only for my own peace of mind.

And yet.

Definitive statements are hard to make about Lyme disease, since much of our understanding of this illness and the organism(s) that cause it is built on a foundation of shifting sands.

The more I learn about Lyme, the less I feel I know about it. Questions don't lead to answers; they only lead to more questions. Every time I think I've nailed down one aspect of the disease, I come across information that seems to contradict everything I've learned, forcing me to decide whether what I've just read matches my experience or is completely off base. And if I decide it's off base, is that because I'm not really suffering from Lyme disease at all, but from relapsing tick fever instead (or in tandem)? More intriguingly, could it be because the researchers themselves are suffering from cultural or personal biases that are skewing what should be objective findings?

Don't think it doesn't happen. Bias long ago replaced dispassionate reasoning in the field of scientific research. You only have to read a handful of papers to discover that. And I've read so much more than a handful of papers.

Way back when my diagnostic misadventure first began, I remember feeling as though I'd been handed a puzzle with a critical piece missing.

I still feel that way.

Six years down the road, I can't tell you with any degree of certainty the name of the organism(s) that infiltrated my body, causing such tremendous upheaval. The name of the illness, on the other hand, is most certainly borreliosis, regardless of specific species of bacteria that gave rise to it. Neuroborreliosis (the name given to borreliosis when it infects the brain) may be the better word.

You can call it Lyme disease, if you think you can make that illness fit.

You can call it relapsing tick fever, if you'd rather.

You can call it both.

I'm not sure I care much any more.

My search for answers is more on an academic level these days.

Sanity dictates that approach.

For all the rocks I've turned over — and the many I've hit — I'm not at all sure I'm getting any closer to the answers I'm seeking. I'm not even sure that I'm asking the right questions — nor am I convinced that researchers are asking the right questions either — but I'm willing to keep asking them until I can think up better ones.

And with better questions will inevitably come better answers.

Someday.

When I was first diagnosed in 2007, I was informed that I was the index case for Lyme disease in my area, which means that I was the first person in my small town ever to have her case of Lyme disease officially confirmed.

It's never good to be a medical pioneer.

You can forget clinical expertise.

In its absence, treatment is delivered via the prevailing guidelines. Not only did those guidelines recommend against treating with antibiotics beyond one month, but public health officials in this country were actively publishing articles in medical journals and making public statements warning doctors and patients alike against the use of long-term antibiotics in the treatment of Lyme. That authorities were also going after the one doctor willing to treat me according to the ILADS guidelines was just the icing on the cake.

The well had been thoroughly poisoned.

That another doctor would offer to send me to someone for long-term antibiotics a year later reflected a growing unease within the medical profession over how Lyme disease is being handled in this country.

Maybe I should've taken the advice of the doctor I met through improper channels and left the country in pursuit of treatment, but I refused to leave my home and incur massive medical bills in a foreign country because the healthcare system in this country couldn't get its act together. It still can't. And I still refuse to leave.

Fortunately the situation has gotten easier for at least some Lyme sufferers in Canada. In 2009, British Columbia cleared the way for naturopaths to start prescribing antibiotics, so now anyone with Lyme in this province can get antibiotic treatment without having to deal with medical doctors. While they still have to leave the healthcare system and pay countless thousands of dollars for their treatment, at least they can now get long-term antibiotics without being made to feel like criminals.

I count myself among the lucky ones who managed to find a naturopath who proved to be more than up to the challenge of treating me for an entrenched Lyme infection. That naturopath was not located in British Columbia and therefore wasn't able to treat me with antibiotics (and likely wouldn't have even if it had been an option). But he had known me for many years. He knew the person I was before Lyme entered my life and was determined that I would one day be that person again.

Lyme patients with advanced infections who are unwilling to work with a naturopath in place of a medical doctor continue to be without options within Canada unless they can find some way to get that treatment while remaining under the radar.

So what will it take for them to get those options?

Quite possibly it'll take government intervention.

Several American states have either passed or are contemplating legislation allowing doctors to treat entrenched Lyme disease infections as they see fit without fear of disciplinary action, recognizing that a division in medical opinion exists, that there are merits on both sides of the argument, and that it'll likely be a very long time before that division goes away. Electing to follow the ILADS guidelines (which advocates the use of long-term oral and IV antibiotics, depending on stage) instead of the IDSA guidelines (which doesn't) does not in and of itself constitute a failure to provide appropriate medical care.

So far, no such legislation has been enacted in Canada, but many are calling for it. Forget for a moment that it's never a good idea to let politicians muck around in medical care. They do that anyway. The bigger problem that must be addressed is that when you drive the treatment of a medical condition underground, you create a potentially dangerous situation for which there are no real controls.

Nobody wants that.

Legislation may be the only way out of it.
Unless cooler heads prevail.
And there aren't many cool heads in this game.

THE MISSING PIECE OF THE PUZZLE

For everything that's known about Lyme disease, there are still an extraordinary number of unknowns in some fairly fundamental areas.

Researchers can't say for certain exactly how Bb makes people sick, although they can see quite clearly that it does. And they don't know nearly as much about the genetics and physiology of Bb as they would like to, even though they long ago succeeded in mapping its genome. They also don't know for certain why some people continue to have symptoms after what should've been successful antibiotic treatment. The survival forms that I mention in this book are the explanation that makes the most sense to me, but not everyone agrees with that viewpoint.

Even if everyone did agree, researchers still can't say what percentage of Canadians have Lyme disease or how many have co-infections with other tick-borne illnesses, an area woefully lacking in research. They certainly don't know how many strains of Bb are at play in Canada, how many novel species of borrelia are present in this country, and which, if any, cause illness in humans. They also don't know the full range of creatures acting as reservoirs for Bb infections in Canada and they can't say with any degree of certainty how many different tick species carry the bacteria, since little research has been done on vectors other than *Ixodes scapularis*, *Ixodes pacificus* and *Ixodes angustus*.

That's a whole lot of Ixodes. But when you consider how many species of ticks have been shown to carry Lyme bacteria south of the border and when you consider that many of those also make their homes in Canada or find their way here on the bodies of migrating birds, it's a drop in the bucket.

And that's not all.

Researchers don't know the full scope of where in the Canadian landscape Lyme is making its home these days. I mean, they imply that they do — they confidently list endemic regions on their maps and even create computer models to show where Lyme-infected ticks will likely spread in the coming years — and yet there are a plethora of Lyme sufferers who have already contracted the illness in areas not listed as being endemic, which would seem to suggest they're all victims of adventitious ticks.

It's estimated that between 3 and 4.5 billion songbirds migrate into Canada every spring with more arriving during fall migration. It's further been estimated that those cheerful little birds could be carrying anywhere up to 175 million *Ixodes scapularis* ticks into the country each year, most of which are nymphs. That's a lot of ticks. And that's just one tick species of the dozens known to harbour Bb.

So then perhaps all of these people are contracting Lyme disease from adventitious ticks that are being carried outside endemic regions by birds, something that would mean that adventitious ticks are playing a far greater role in human infection than they've traditionally been given credit for. The other option is that endemic regions are far more widespread than researchers realize and may very well include many areas that don't currently make it onto official maps, something that's quite likely when you consider how little active surveillance has been undertaken in Canada. Clearly there's a need for more research.

But the problem is deeper than simply a lack of research. Lyme is a disease that, almost forty years after it was first identified, still doesn't have a universally accepted definition and it doesn't look like one will be arriving anytime soon. Is Lyme best defined as infection with Bb and only Bb or does that definition need to be opened up to include other borrelia species? Does the definition need to include possible co-infections with unrelated organisms, some of which can dramatically alter the clinical picture, making Lyme both more severe and harder to defeat? Do Lyme disease and relapsing tick fever need to be merged into a single illness that can sometimes present with an EM rash, at other times with remitting/recurring fevers, and at still other times with neither? Does it need to be broadened even further than that?

Or does the definition need to be changed entirely? Maybe, for instance, Bb is not the actual cause of Lyme disease but rather a common co-infecting organism that's been wrongly accused of causing Lyme disease in much the same way that sow bugs get wrongfully accused of causing injury to living plant material when in reality they show up once the damage has been done by something else, the real attacker seeing wisdom in remaining hidden.

Wouldn't that be ironic? The suggestion itself is blasphemous. But then maybe a little blasphemy is just what this situation is calling for.

The divisions in the scientific community are simply too wide and too contentious for consensus to be reached on even such a fundamental issue as the disease's definition, and without a working definition, it's hard to imagine how many of the other issues surrounding Lyme can be adequately resolved.

Which leads to the farce we have now.

I don't know why my illness started with a trip to the dentist and I admit that it was a strange place to begin this tale. Any other writer would surely have skipped over that troubling anecdote in an effort to streamline one of the few aspects of this story that could easily be streamlined.

Don't mention it and it didn't happen.

Voilà.

But the strange way this debacle started is part of what continues to perplex me.

I've read other people's stories.

I've listened to their anecdotes.

So I know that I'm not the first person to suddenly fall ill with Lyme when there was nothing in the days and weeks leading up to its abrupt onset to suggest that anything was amiss. Sure, there may have been hints that something wasn't 100 percent right — unexplained fatigue or emotional outbursts with no apparent trigger — but nothing to suggest I was about to go down hard and stay down for many years.

I suppose that's just part of the quirky nature of this disease.

Also a part of its quirky nature are the reports that some Lyme sufferers are plagued by lucid dreams, horrific nightmares, or imagery so vivid that the vividness itself is alarming. Others, like me, report the loss of the ability to dream.

Eventually my dreams came back, but only after a five-year hiatus. I don't know what brought them back. One day my subconscious simply awoke, as if from a coma, and started spewing some of the most dazzling, perplexing brain puzzles I can ever remember experiencing.

I hope someday to figure a few of them out. I hope someday to figure a lot of things out. I hope someday arrives soon.

Mostly I just hope.

SALVATION ARMY

Lyme disease may not have killed me, but it certainly put an end to life as I knew it.

I used to run an information technology company with my husband. I remember that like an explorer remembers a desert mirage, wafting in and out of view, never quite in focus. Within months of my experiencing my first Lyme symptoms, my husband was forced to run the company alone and when he wasn't busy doing that, he was doing the cooking, the cleaning, the shopping and the laundry. He closed doors that I inexplicably left hanging wide open. Turned off burners set on high. Tied my shoelaces when my fingers no longer knew the routine. He picked me up off floors and on those rare occasions when I left the house, he reminded me where I was, why I was there, and who in God's name I was talking to. He chauffeured me to emergency rooms, doctor appointments, and wherever I needed to go for medical tests, even when such efforts meant ten-hour drives. And he tried, with his fully functional brain, to understand why doctors were doing their absolute best to be such useless tools.

And sometimes he left. The endless suffering was just too much, so he took refuge in the company of friends and strangers alike. Yet although he'd sometimes leave, he always came back, and I have to confess that if the situation were reversed, I'm not sure I would've done the same.

I wouldn't have done the same. I know the darkness in my own soul well enough to know that when a situation calls for an extreme of human compassion, I fall far short of the mark every time.

✳

I owe an enormous debt of gratitude to N. Richard Pragnell, ND, DC, HD, HDMS, for walking into the middle of a desperate situation and doing everything in his power to turn this cruel disease back on itself. It was an awesome thing to witness. Unlike the parade of medical doctors who found themselves blinking in the headlights of a disease they could not or would not understand, this experienced naturopath not only recognized the severity of the situation, he took decisive action to slay the beast that was doing its best to slay me.

He never faltered in his conviction that we would one day win this battle. Even when my own conviction faltered badly. Even when I was face down on the bathroom floor begging to be killed. Even when the afterlife seemed nearer to me than the present one.

He met every challenge with creativity and compassion. He introduced me to a wide array of treatments, the likes of which I'd never before encountered. More importantly, he wasn't afraid to look things up or consult with colleagues as far away as Germany in his efforts to develop the course of treatment that we continue to hope will one day eradicate this disease.

Without his help, I would not have survived. That's a debt I can never repay.

Before Lyme came into my life, I would never have considered battling a major illness without the help of a medical doctor. Now I sidestep conventional healthcare as much as possible in favor of a system of medicine that strikes me as a little more sane. It took a lot to change my way of thinking. It took a cataclysm.

It also took an army to get me on my feet again. A coalition of the willing.

Many people played crucial roles in restoring my tick-shattered life to something I could recognize as my own. My husband and my naturopath deserve the lion's share of the credit since they did the most to help me and since — let's be honest here — they found themselves on the receiving end of some fairly offensive behavior. No one will ever accuse me of being a saint in times of great distress.

Yet they weren't alone in their efforts.

I also received help from a chiropractor, a registered massage therapist, a physiotherapist, a speech-language pathologist, a psychologist, and a neuropsychologist. Friends, neighbors, family, and even total strangers who heard about my plight came to me with suggestions for how to restore my health. I permitted a medical doctor with expertise in Lyme disease to consult on my case whenever I found myself confronted with a baffling circumstance, but that's all he was permitted to do. My faith in conventional medicine had been shattered to the extent that allowing a medical doctor to play any significant role in my treatment was out of the question.

It still is.

SELECTED BIBLIOGRAPHY

Abele, D., and K. Anders. 1990. *The many faces and phases of borreliosis in Lyme disease.* J Am Acad Dermatol. 23(2):167-86.

Aberer, E., and P. Duray. 1991. *Morphology of Borrelia burgdorferi: Structural patterns of cultured borreliae in relation to staining methods.* J Clin Microbiol. 29(4):764-72

Aguero-Rosenfeld, M., et al. 2005. *Diagnosis of Lyme borreliosis.* J Clin Microbiol. 18(3):484-509.

Ang, C., D. Notermans, and M. Hommes. 2011. *Large differences between test strategies for the detection of anti-borrelia antibodies are revealed by comparing eight ELISAs and five immunoblots.* Eur J Clin Microbiol Infect Dis. 30:1027-1032.

Anguita, J., C. Olson, Jr., and E. Fikrig. *"Immune responses to spirochetes": Clinical Immunology: Principles and practice.* Edited by Robert R. Rich, et al. Third Edition. Mosby/Elsevier Saunders, Inc., 2008.

Banerjee, S., et al. 1992. *Seroprevalence survey of borreliosis in children with chronic arthritis in British Columbia, Canada.* J Rheumatol. 19(10):1620-4.

Banerjee, S., et al. 1998. *Tick-borne relapsing fever in British Columbia, Canada: First isolation of Borrelia hermsii.* J Clin Microbiol. 36(12):3505-3508.

Barbour, Alan G. *Lyme Disease: The Cause, the Cure, the Controversy.* Baltimore and London: Johns Hopkins University Press, 1996.

Barbour, A. *"Relapsing Fever and Other Borrelia Diseases": Tropical Infectious Diseases.* Edited by Richard L. Guerrant, et al. Second Edition. Philadelphia: Churchill Livingstone, 2006.

Bean, Constance A. *Beating Lyme: Understanding and Treating This Complex and Often Misdiagnosed Disease.* New York: AMACOM, 2008.

Betkowski, Bev. *Getting a grip on ticks in Alberta.* Faculty of Agricultural Life and Environmental Sciences, University of Alberta. Press release: July 12, 2012. Downloaded from University of Alberta website: July 13, 2012.

BC Centre for Disease Control. *British Columbia 2007 Annual Summary of Reportable Diseases.* Provincial Health Services Authority. November, 2008. Available from: www.bccdc.ca

BC Centre for Disease Control. *British Columbia 2008 Annual Summary of Reportable Diseases.* Provincial Health Services Authority. July 31, 2009. Available from: www.bccdc.ca

BC Centre for Disease Control. *British Columbia 2009 Annual Summary of Reportable Diseases.* Provincial Health Services Authority. August 18, 2010. Available from: www.bccdc.ca

BC Centre for Disease Control. *British Columbia 2010 Annual Summary of Reportable Diseases.* Provincial Health Services Authority. June 28, 2012. Available from: www.bccdc.ca

Bratton, R., et al. 2008. *Diagnosis and treatment of Lyme disease.* Mayo Clinic Proc. 83(5):566-71.

Brisson, D., et al. 2011. *Biodiversity of Borrelia burgdorferi strains in tissues of Lyme disease patients.* PLoS ONE 6(8):e22926.

British Ecological Society. *Predicting the spread of ticks across Canada.* ScienceDaily (www.sciencedaily.com). Posted: March 5, 2012. Accessed: March 6, 2012.

Brorson, O. and S. Brorson. 1997. *Transformation of cystic forms of Borrelia burgdorferi to normal, mobile spirochetes.* Infection. 25(4):240-246.

Buhner, Stephen Harrod. *Healing Lyme: Natural Healing and Prevention of Lyme Borreliosis and Its Co-infections.* Randolph, Vermont: Raven Press, 2005.

Bunikis, J. and A. Barbour. 2005. *Third borrelia species in white-footed mice.* Emerg Infect Dis. 11(7):1150-1151.

Bunikis, J., et al. 2004. *Typing of borrelia relapsing fever group strains.* Emerg Infect Dis. 10(9):1661-1664.

Burgdorfer, W. 1999. *Keynote address — The complexity of vector-borne spirochetes (Borrelia spp.).* 12th International Conference on Lyme Disease and Other Spirochetal and Tick-Borne Disorders. Posted on CBC website (www.cbc.ca). Accessed: December 25, 2007.

Burrascano, Joseph J., Jr. *Advanced Topics in Lyme Disease: Diagnostic Hints and Treatment Guidelines for Lyme and Other Tick Borne Illnesses.* Fifteenth Edition. Bethesda, Maryland: International Lyme and Associated Diseases Society, 2005.

Cadavid, D., *"Spirochetal Infections": Bacterial Infections of the Central Nervous System: Handbook of Clinical Neurology.* Edited by Karen L. Roos and Allan R. Tunkel. Amsterdam: Elsevier, 2010. pp. 179-219.

Canadian Public Health Laboratory Network Guidelines. 2007. *The laboratory diagnosis of Lyme borreliosis: Guidelines from the Canadian Public Health Laboratory Network.* Can J Infect Dis Med Mircobiol. 18(2):145-148.

Carpi G., et al. 2011. *Metagenomic profile of the bacterial communities associated with Ixodes ricinus ticks.* PLoS ONE 6(10):e25604.

CBC Radio One. *IDEAS: The Bacteria Revolution.* CBC website (www.cbc.ca/ideas/feaures/shows/bacteria/bacttext.html). Aired: Friday, May 28 & June 4, 1999, 9:05 p.m. Accessed online: December 25, 2007.

Chaconas, G. 2012. *CSM Murray Award Lecture — Functional studies of the Lyme disease spirochete — from molecules to mice.* Can J. Microbiol. 58:236-248.

Cutler, Sally J. *"Relapsing Fever Borrelia": Molecular Medical Microbiology.* Edited by Max Sussman. London: Academic Press, 2002.

Dresser A., P. Hardy and G. Chaconas. 2009. *Investigation of the genes involved in antigenic switching at the vlsE locus in Borrelia burgdorferi: An essential role for the RuvAB branch migrase.* PLoS Pathog. 5(12):e1000680.

Dworkin, M., et al. 1998. *Tick-borne relapsing fever in the Northwestern United States and Southwestern Canada.* Clinical Infectious Diseases. 26:122-31.

Dworkin, M., et al. 2002. *The epidemiology of tick-borne relapsing fever in the United States.* Am J Trop Med Hyg. 66(6):753-758.

Edlow, Jonathon. *Bull's Eye: Unravelling the Medical Mystery of Lyme.* New Haven and London: Yale University Press, 2004.

Favaro, Avis. *Lyme disease experts fear disease explosion.* CTV News (www.ctvnews.ca). Posted: June 20, 2012. Accessed: July 6, 2012.

Fayerman, P. *Most B.C. doctors not trained to diagnose Lyme disease.* Vancouver Sun. Posted: March 29, 2011.

Fihn, S. and E. Larson. 1980. *Tick-borne relapsing fever in the Pacific Northwest: An under-diagnosed illness?* West J Med. 133:203-209.

Funk, Rebekah. *B.C. funds study of fibromyalgia, Lyme disease, chronic fatigue.* The Globe and Mail (www.theglobeandmail.com). Posted: March 30, 2011.

Grainger, Lia. *Lyme and the tale of two tests.* National Post (www.nationalpost.com). Posted: August 5, 2009. Accessed: August 6, 2009

Health Canada. 2012. *Lyme disease test kits and limitations.* Canadian Adverse Reaction Newsletter. 22(4):1.

Hearle, E. 1934. *Vectors of relapsing fever in relation to an outbreak of the disease in British Columbia.* Can Med Assoc J. 30:494-497.

Henry, B. and M. Morshed. 2011. *Lyme disease in British Columbia: Are we really missing an epidemic?* BCMJ. 53(5):224–229.

Henry, B., A. Crabtree and M. Morshed. 2011. *Physician awareness of Lyme disease in British Columbia.* BCMJ. 53(2).

Henry, B., et al. 2012. *Lyme disease: Knowledge, beliefs, and practices of physicians in a low-endemic area.* Canadian Family Physician. 58(5):e289-e295.

Karlen, Arno. *Biography of a Germ.* New York: Anchor Books, 2000.

Koomey, M. 1997. *Bacterial pathogenesis: A variation on variation in Lyme disease.* Current Biology. 7:R538-R540.

Lange, W., T. Schwan, J. Frame. 1991. *Can protracted relapsing fever resemble Lyme disease?* Medical Hypotheses. 35(2):77-79.

Leighton, P., et al. 2012. *Predicting the speed of tick invasion: An empirical model of range expansion for Lyme disease vector Ixodes scapularis in Canada.* Journal of Applied Ecology. 49(2):457-464.

Levi, Taal, et al. 2012. *Deer, predators, and the emergence of Lyme disease.* PNAS. 2012:1-6.

Liang, F., et al. 2002. *An immune evasion mechanism for spirochetal persistence in Lyme borreliosis.* J Exp Med. 195(4):415-422.

Lim, L. and J. Rosenbaum. 2006. *Borrelia hermsii causing relapsing fever and uveitis.* American Journal of Ophthalmology. 142(2):348-349.

Lopez, J., et al. 2010. *A novel surface antigen of relapsing fever spirochetes can discriminate between relapsing fever and Lyme borreliosis.* Clin Vaccine Immunol. 17(4):564-571.

MacDonald, A. 2008. *Biofilm of Borrelia burgdorferi and clinical implications for chronic borreliosis.* University of New Haven Lyme Disease Symposium, New Haven Connecticut.

Mak, S., M. Morshed, and B. Henry. 2010. *Ecological niche modeling of Lyme disease in British Columbia, Canada.* Journal of Medical Entomology. 47(1):99-102.

McNeil, Donald G. *New tick-borne disease is discovered.* The New York Times. September 19, 2011. p. D6.

Miklossy, J., et al. 2008. *Persisting atypical and cystic forms of Borrelia burgdorferi and local inflammation in Lyme neuroborreliosis.* Journal of Neuroinflammation. 5:40.

Montgomery, R. and S. Malawista. 1994. *Borrelia burgdorferi and the macrophage: Routine annihilation but occasional haven?* Parasitology Today. 10(4):154-157.

Moriarty, T., et al. 2008. *Real-time high resolution 3D imaging of the Lyme disease spirochete adhering to and escaping from the vasculature of a living host.* PLoS Pathog. 4(6):e1000090.

Morshed, M. 1999. *Tick-borne diseases and laboratory diagnosis.* CMPT Connections. 3(1):1-2.

Morshed, M., et al. 2006. *Distribution and characterization of Borrelia burgdorferi isolates from Ixodes scapularis and presence in mammalian host in Ontario, Canada.* J Med Entomol. 43(4):762-73.

Ogden, N., et al. 2006. *Ixodes scapularis ticks collected by passive surveillance in Canada: Analysis of geographic distribution and infection with Lyme borreliosis agent Borrelia burgdorferi.* J Med Entomol. 43(3):600-609.

Ogden, N., et al. 2008. *Lyme Disease: A zoonotic disease of increasing importance to Canadians.* Canadian Family Physician. 54:1381-1384.

Ogden, N., et al. 2008. *Risk maps for range expansion of the Lyme disease vector, Ixodes scapularis, in Canada now and with climate change.* International Journal of Health Geographic Services. 7:24.

Ogden, N., et al. 2008. *Role of migratory birds in introduction and range expansion of Ixodes scapularis ticks and of Borrelia burgdorferi and Anaplasma phagocytophilum in Canada.* Appl Environ Mircobiol. 74(6):1780-90.

Ogden, N., et al. 2008. *The rising challenge of Lyme borreliosis in Canada.* Public Health Agency of Canada. Canada Communicable Disease Report. 34(1).

Ogden, N., et al. 2009. *The emergence of Lyme in Canada.* CMAJ. 180(12):1221-1224.

Ogden, N., et al. 2010. *Active and passive surveillance and phylogenetic analysis of Borrelia burgdorferi elucidate the process of Lyme disease risk emergence in Canada.* Environ Health Perspect. 118(7):909-914.

Ogden, N., et al. 2011. *Investigation of genotypes of Borrelia burgdorferi in Ixodes scapularis ticks collected in surveillance in Canada.* Appl Environ Microbio. 77(10):3244-54.

Ostfeld, Richard S. *Lyme Disease: The Ecology of a Complex System.* New York: Oxford University Press, 2011.

Palmer, J. and D. Crawford. 1933. *Relapsing tick fever in North America, with a report of an outbreak in British Columbia.* Can Med Assoc J. 28:643-7.

Platanov, A., et al. 2011. *Humans infected with relapsing fever spirochete Borrelia miyamotoi, Russia.* Emerg Infect Dis. 17(10):1816-1823.

Province of British Columbia. *Public Health Act.* Victoria, BC: Crown Publications, Queens Printer. Consolidation Date: October 27, 2010.

Putteet-Driver, A., J. Zhong, and A. Barbour. 2004. *Transgenic expression of RecA of the spirochetes Borrelia burgdorferi and Borrelia hermsii in Escherichis coli revealed differences in DNA repair and recombination phenotypes.* Journal of Bacteriology. 186(8):2262-2274

Reik, L., W. Burgodorfer, and J. Donaldson. 1986. *Neurologic abnormalities in Lyme disease without Erythema Chronicum Migrans.* The American Journal of Medicine. 81:73-78.

Ricks, Delthia. *Tick-borne virus, new to Americas, identified in Missouri.* The Korea Herald (nwww.koreaherald.com). Posted: September 6, 2012.

Rosner, Bryan. *The Top 10 Lyme Disease Treatments.* Lake Tahoe: BioMed Publishing Group, 2007.

Sapi, E., et al. 2012. *Characterization of biofilm formation by Borrelia burgdorferi in vitro.* PLOS One 7(10):e48227.

Schmidt, Brian T. *Chronic Lyme Disease in British Columbia: A Review of Strategic and Policy Issues.* Vancouver, BC: British Columbia Provincial Health Services Authority, 2010.

Schwan, T., et al. 1996. *G1pQ: An antigen for serological discrimination between relapsing fever and Lyme borreliosis.* Journal of Clinical Microbiology. 34(10):2483-2492.

Scott, J., and L. Durden. 2009. *First isolation of Lyme disease spirochete, Borrelia burgdorferi, from ticks collected from songbirds in Ontario, Canada.* North American Bird Bander. 34(3):97-101.

Scott, J., et al. 2010. *Detection of Lyme disease spirochete, Borrelia burgdorferi sensu lato, including three novel genotypes in ticks (Acari: Ixodidae) collected from songbirds (Passeriformes) across Canada.* Journal of Vector Ecology. 35(1):124-139.

Scott, J., J. Anderson and L. Durden. 2012. *Widespread dispersal of Borrelia burgdorferi-infected ticks collected from songbirds across Canada.* Journal of Parasitology. 98(1):49-59.

Sperling, J., and F. Sperling. 2009. *Lyme borreliosis in Canada: Biological diversity and diagnostic complexity from an entomological perspective.* The Canadian Entomologist. 141(6):521-549.

Sperling, J., et al. 2012. *Evolving perspectives on Lyme borreliosis in Canada.* The Open Neurology Journal. 6(Suppl. 1-M4):94-103.

Spiller, G. 1986. *Tick-borne relapsing fever due to Borrelia hermsii in British Columbia.* Can Med Assoc J. 134:46-7.

Stafford, K. *Tick Management Handbook.* Bulletin no. 1010. Rev. ed. New Haven, Connecticut: The Connecticut Agricultural Experimental Station, 2007.

Sterngold, John. *Living with Lyme: Bacterium can 'cloak' itself.* The Willits News (http://www.willitsnews.com/). Posted: September 30, 2009. Accessed October 6, 2009.

Sterngold, John. *Living with Lyme: A phenomenally complex disease.* The Willits News (http://www.willitsnews.com/). Posted: November 4, 2009. Accessed: November 5, 2009.

Stevenson, B. 2001. *Borrelia burgdorferi: A (somewhat) clonal bacterial species.* Trends in Microbiology. 9(10):471.

Stonehouse, A., J. Studdiford and C. Henry. 2010. *An update on the diagnosis and treatment of early Lyme disease: "Focusing on the bull's eye, you may miss the mark."* J Emerg Med. 39(5):e147-151.

Tauber, S., et al. 2011. *Long-term intrathecal infusion of outer surface protein C from Borrelia burgdorferi causes axonal damage.* Journal of Neuropathy & Experimental Neurology. 70(9):748-757.

Teng, J., et al. 2011. *Prevalence of tick-borne pathogens in the South Okanagan, British Columbia: Active surveillance in ticks (Dermacentor andersonii) and deer mice (Peromyscus maniculatus).* BCMJ. 53(3):122-127.

Wormser, G., et al. 2006. *The clinical assessment, treatment and prevention of Lyme disease, human granulocytic anaplasmosis, and babesiosis: Clinical practice guidelines by the Infectious Disease Society of America.* Clin Infect Dis. 2006. 43(1 November):1089-1134.

ILLUSTRATIONS

Page 54
1. Under a high magnification, this scanning electron micrograph depicts three Gram-negative, anaerobic, *Borrelia burgdorferi* bacteria, which had been derived from a pure culture.
CDC Image # 13178, Photo credit: Jamice Haney Carr, Content credit: CDC/ Claudia Molins

2. Using darkfield microscopy technique, this photomicrograph, magnified 400x, reveals the presence of spirochete, or "corkscrew-shaped" bacteria known as *Borrelia burgdorferi*.
CDC Image # 6631, Content credit: CDC

Page 101
The black-legged ticks *Ixodes scapularis* and *Ixodes pacificus*.

1. The black-legged tick *Ixodes scapularis* is found on a wide range of hosts including mammals, birds and reptiles.
CDC Image # 1669, Photo credit: Jim Gathany, Content credit: CDC/ Michael L. Levin, Ph. D.

2. The western black-legged tick, *I. pacificus*, is a known vector for the bacteria *Borrelia burgdorferi*.
CDC Image # 7663, Photo credit: James Gathany, Content credit: CDC/ James Gathany; William Nicholson

Page 111
The life cycle of an *Ixodes scapularis* tick.

Page 131
Erythema migrans rashes
1. This 2007 photograph shows the iconic "bull's-eye" rash long associated with Lyme disease, which manifested at the site of a tick bite on this woman's posterior right upper arm.
CDC Image # 9874, Photo credit: James Gathany, Content credit: CDC

2. This image shows the left thigh of a patient who developed the characteristic red, expanding rash called erythema migrans (EM), caused by the *Borrelia burgdorferi* bacterium.
CDC Image # 14471, Content credit: CDC

3. This image shows right calf of a patient who developed the characteristic red, expanding rash called erythema migrans (EM), caused by the *Borrelia burgdorferi* bacterium.
CDC Image # 14475, Content credit: CDC

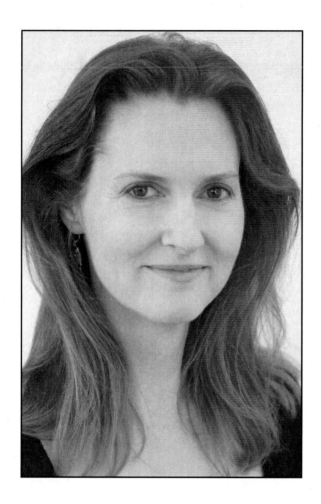

ABOUT THE AUTHOR

Vanessa Farnsworth has published in national and regional publications, including *Canadian Gardening, Canadian Living, Cottage, Garden Making, The Creston Valley Advance, The Grower, Harrowsmith Country Life, Kootenay Life East, Route 3,* and *Vitality Magazine.* She holds a degree in English from Toronto's York University, a diploma in print journalism from Oakville's Sheridan College, and she studied creative writing at The Humber School for Writers. Her literary fiction has been published in journals across Canada and in the United States, including *The Dalhousie Review, dANDelion, The New Quarterly, PRECIPICe, Qwerty,* and *Reed Magazine.*